Family Fuel:

A Busy Mom's Guide to Healthy Living for the Family

Getting Back to Basics and
Connecting Through Clean, Healthy Meals

by

Jennifer Wren Tolo, R.N.

DORRANCE PUBLISHING CO
EST. 1920
PITTSBURGH, PENNSYLVANIA 15238

The contents of this work, including, but not limited to, the accuracy of events, people, and places depicted; opinions expressed; permission to use previously published materials included; and any advice given or actions advocated are solely the responsibility of the author, who assumes all liability for said work and indemnifies the publisher against any claims stemming from publication of the work.

All Rights Reserved
Copyright © 2016 by Jennifer Wren Tolo, R.N.

No part of this book may be reproduced or transmitted, downloaded, distributed, reverse engineered, or stored in or introduced into any information storage and retrieval system, in any form or by any means, including photocopying and recording, whether electronic or mechanical, now known or hereinafter invented without permission in writing from the publisher.

Dorrance Publishing Co
585 Alpha Drive
Pittsburgh, PA 15238
Visit our website at *www.dorrancebookstore.com*

ISBN: 978-1-4809-3012-4
eISBN: 978-1-4809-2989-0

Table of Contents

Chapter 1: 1
    Food as Fuel: Why Home Cooking and Family Meals are Keys to Healthy Living

Chapter 2: 9
    Tips on How to Get Your Family to Eat Healthier and Connect

Chapter 3: 19
    Recipes for Healthy Living

Chapter 4: 23
    Tips for Creating Healthy Habits for the Family

Chapter 5: 27
    Elimination Plan: Figuring Out What You May Be Reacting or Sensitive To.

Chapter 6: 31
    Morning Fuel: Breakfast

Chapter 7: 35
    Soups and Vegetables

Chapter 8: 43
    Main Meals

Chapter 9: 53
    Muffins

Chapter 10: 59
    Desserts

Dedication

To my husband, Eric, and my boys, Larson, Ollie, Brodie, and Mathias…

Thank you for keeping me on my path and reminding me why staying strong and riding out the roller coaster ride of life is so worth it in the end! I love you to infinity.

Introduction

I am a firm believer that everything in life happens for a reason. I am blessed to have four children and a wonderful husband who happens to be an open-minded orthopaedic surgeon. When we first got married, I was a critical care nurse, finishing up my Masters in Nursing Administration, thinking I was going to change healthcare through administration. In reality, I became increasingly frustrated with nursing practice, administration, and healthcare. Then I became blessed with four amazing boys, each leading me to be more soulfully and spiritually awakened.

The birth of my first son, Larson, awakened me to grace, selflessness, unconditional love, and a mother's heart. I was roused to my calling and my purpose with the birth of my second son, Ollie, who had a massive neonatal stroke an hour after his birth. My path began to shift from traditional healthcare to alternative and integrated health with the blessing of this tiny little guy. I became Reiki Certified, an American Council on Exercise (ACE) certified personal trainer, and earned my first nutrition certification. Apparently, I was still napping on my spiritual, visionary path as while I was pregnant with my fourth son, Mathias, my third son, Brodie, at two and a half years old, was diagnosed with high-risk acute lymphoblastic leukemia.

As grateful as I am to the hospital for "curing" and ridding Brodie of cancer, they had to take him close to death to do so, killing the diseased cells as well as healthy cells. What shocked me was the doctors and dieticians telling me "just get calories in him" when I asked for nutrition advice. I was astounded, believing that cells need good nutrients in order to grow to be healthy: quality as well as quantity. Yet I watched people with fast food and smiles trying to appease their sick children. I sought out alternatives to this model and found the Institute for Integrative Nutrition, where I became a certified Holistic Health Counselor.

Now, my purpose is clear – to help people heal and live healthy lives through good nutrition, whole foods, self-awareness, responsibility, hope, love, laughter, connecting with self and others, and moving with play and joy. My son is now ten and cancer free. When the nurse practitioner in the well clinic at the hospital where he received his treatment told him what a strong and healthy boy he is, he told her, "It is because of my mom."

My parents blessed me with healthy whole food, sweets, "junk" on the rare occasion, and family meals. Although, like I did as a kid, my boys complain about the scarcity of junk food and family mealtime, I know they will thank me as happy and healthy adults. My son, Brodie, in his comment to his nurse practitioner, gave me the best thank you a boy could! I hope you enjoy this wisdom I have to impart to you. I wish you and your loved ones' health and happiness!

Chapter 1

Food as Fuel

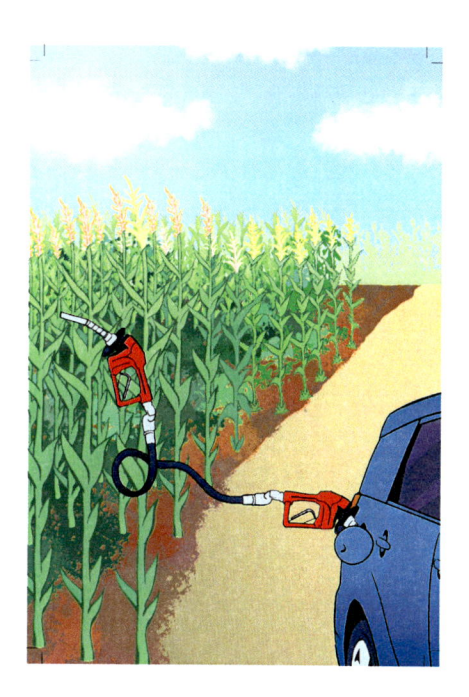

In all of my experiences as a mom and a health professional giving workshops to schools, communities and families, the main message I strive to convey is this: food is fuel for our bodies, and our body and brain performance is reliant on the type, amount and quality of that fuel.

Although we are meant to enjoy the experience of eating—the flavors, textures and smells—the eating experience can become emotional and psychological in its connection to people, nostalgia, festivities, and family. We get into trouble as a nation of fast paced, quick fix, "make it easy because I do not have time" people when we stop paying attention to the quality of the fuel and how we fuel our bodies. We use food as a reward instead of as energy and often mindlessly eat, having no connection to taste, hunger and satiety.

We often forgo the process of sitting down as a family and eating/ digesting our food slowly for a more mindless, distracted, and disconnected process where we consume more, and we do not connect to the fuel for our bodies.

A report from the USDA survey, *What We Eat in America Survey*, found that we are snacking more now than ever. Ninety-seven percent of Americans reported snacking at least once a day, 82 percent reported snacking two times a day, and 56 percent of American's had three or more snacks a day (USDA 2014a). The Hartman Group, a consumer research company, attributes this rise in snacking to factors such as less time meal planning, skipping meals, and a diminished concept of family meals, as well as people eating alone more (Hartman Group, 2013). Food consumption has increased in America, particularly with snacking, however Americans seem more disconnected with food, mindlessly eating, often on the go and with others preparing the food, be it a restaurant or processed food manufacturer.

Shifting our focus from food as a reward or an afterthought to food as vital fuel for our bodies and brains will go a long way towards improving the overall health of our nation. Taking time to slow down, enjoy, and connect with our food is a key part of this. A study from the *American College of Clinical Nutrition* (2011) found that participants who chewed each bite of food forty times consumed 12 percent less calories than those that chewed fifteen times (Li et al, 2011). So there is something to be said for sitting at a table, unplugged, and talking as a family, connecting. This allows us to focus on the flavors, the textures, and our bodies' messages that we are full. According to a study in the *American Journal of Preventive Medicine*, watching TV was linked to higher consumption of high calorie, low nutrient food and drink with low amounts of fruit and vegetables in the diet for both adults and children (Pearson and Biddle, 2011). This is the mindlessness of eating, plugged in and focused on external stimuli versus your body and nourishing your body while heeding its messages when full.

In helping my parents move in their retirement, I discovered an old cookbook of my mother's called *"The Seasonal Kitchen: A Return to Fresh Foods"* by Perla Meyers. This was published in 1973, the year I was born! Even back then, we were trumpeting using fresh, seasonal, and local ingredients. That was before microwaves and technology took over our lives in the 1980s. Those days were the meat and potatoes, family sit down meals, but they often lacked variety and fresh, seasonal ingredients. The shift back to fresh, local ingredients and whole food, plant-based diets is upon us now, based on the environmental consciousness (going green) and rising health issues related to preventable diseases and obesity. According to the Center for Disease Control, in 2008, overall medical expenses related to obesity were thought to be more than $147 billion. Medical costs for obese people were $1,429 higher than normal weight individuals. The percentage of Americans with a BMI (Body Mass Index) above twenty-five, signaling overweight, doubled between 1980 and 2000. Americans eat 57 percent more meat today than back in the 1950s, along with 18 percent more whole wheat flour and four times the amount of cheese. Our sweeteners are now mainly corn based instead of from sugar beets, cane sugar, honey, or maple syrup. (Dr. Andrew Weil, "Our Changing Diet," *Self Healing*, August 2014). The bottom line is that, although there is famine in our world, Americans eat literally over a ton per year more than necessary to fuel our bodies and brains. And a good deal of this consumption is done mindlessly, distracted by work, media, or electronics and driven by the processed food industry (watch the movie *Fed Up*). It is time to slow down and connect to our families, our food and our health. As parents, we need to show our children through our example how to live a healthy, happy lifestyle utilizing moderation, mindful decision making about food choices and listening to our bodies' messages regarding how the foods make us feel.

Cooking healthy meals for you and your family does not need to take a great deal of time or money. A Harvard School of Public Health study published online in the BMJ Open (December, 2013) showed that the healthiest diet costs only $1.50 more per day than the least healthy diets. Most meals in this cookbook take twenty minutes or less to prepare. The keys to quick, efficient, healthy meals are: **planning ahead, having a well-stocked pantry, and sometimes prep work in a chunk of time you have earlier in the day or week.**

Cooking is a way to be creative, be connected, and be healthy. YOU choose what you put in your meals and which grain, which vegetable, and which protein to incorporate in it. Having kids have a say in what you cook, maybe even participate in the preparation, will actually help connect them to the food, and they will be more likely to try it. Plus, they gain a tool in their toolbox for life.

We need to be conscious of the messages we send around food. So many people tend to pass on messages of negativity towards food: "you're going to get fat," "that's bad for you," "gluten free," "high protein," "sugar free," "low carb…" What we need to impart to kids is not fear of food, but connection with food as fuel and the "stoplight" philosophy of eating: green foods are "go" foods, yellow foods are "slow down and watch portions," while red foods are "stop—don't eat every day, and just a small amount." The colors represent what colors on a stoplight represent and do not necessarily correlate with the actual color of the food. (*See chart at the end of this chapter.) This helps kids be mindful of their choices instead of fearful of getting fat or sick.

I saw a quote from Dr. Mark Hyman, Director of the Institute for Functional Medicine in Lennox, MA, stating, "We need to stop focusing on counting calories and start focusing on counting chemicals in our food." Let's face it, as an adult, the "forbidden food" is often what we crave or binge on. Adults have trouble self-regulating around food. How can we expect our kids, in a food environment wrought with unhealthy, nutrient scarce, "hyper palatable" rich foods, to make healthy choices that fuel the brain and body? The food industry and food environment, instead, lead them to choices that derail the body's homeostasis mechanisms and bring about disease and disorder? (Hyperpalatables are things that make food taste good, like fat, salt and sugar). Instead, we need to have exposure and allow (in small amounts) foods that may appeal to us, while teaching healthy choices. This way we do not feel deprived, causing us to crave or binge, and we learn moderation.

Dr. Mark Hyman also states that, "Sugar is a recreational drug—it is ok to have a little, but we need to be careful how much and how often." I must add that there are some health conditions, and problems with dopamine system/moderation (the pleasure/reward center of brain), that do require stricter guidelines and limitation around food, but, in general, the 80/20 rule should apply: 80 percent of the time eat whole foods, low in sugar, minimally processed, home cooked while 20 percent of the time, it is ok to indulge in a craving, sweet, salty, meal out... just in moderation. The best thing you can do for your kids is to have healthy options available for snacking: fruits in a bowl on the table, cut up veggies in fridge, and even yogurt, hard boiled eggs, and nuts. Keep higher sugar and higher fat foods put away (homemade ideally) and not always available/stocked.

Send a positive message about food and help create a healthy "Food as Fuel" versus "Food as Reward" relationship. I teach kids fiber equals full. Higher fiber and protein rich foods take longer for the body to digest, so they fuel the body longer than processed, broken-down carbohydrates and sugary foods. A study in the *Journal of Nutrition* by Leidy et. al. (Leidy et., 2015) found that adolescents given a high protein snack versus a high fat snack or no snack in the morning reported longer period of satiety and tended to choose healthier snacks in the afternoon. Choose your fuel carefully and be aware of what, why, and when you are eating.

As a mother of four boys, I know how challenging cooking for your family can be, especially with picky eaters. Did you know it could take up to fifteen exposures to a food before a child can determine if they like something or not? I encourage you to NOT become a short order cook in the family kitchen. Engage your family in the food planning and prep. Ask your kids what veggie they want, maybe offer a few choices. If your kids are hungry, they will eat. They may go on strike until they figure out that this meal you prepared is all there is to eat. They are resilient and smart. Eventually, they will try the meal and a little more the next one.

Occupational therapists working with autistic kids and "sensory" kids recommend slow and steady with introducing new foods. Step 1: place the new food item on the plate to get your child used to seeing it. After a few days or even weeks, step 2: the child may touch it, smell it or even touch tongue to it. After a time, step 3: the child will taste it and decide like or dislike. It is not easy, but the reward and health benefits are HUGE. We need to get kids OFF of the children's menu and on to variety and colors other than yellow and white. I know it is not easy, but we are investing in their long term health and habits, so it is so worth the time and effort now. Variety is SO important because foods give you different nutrients and help expand your taste buds. Varying the color varies the nutrients you receive.

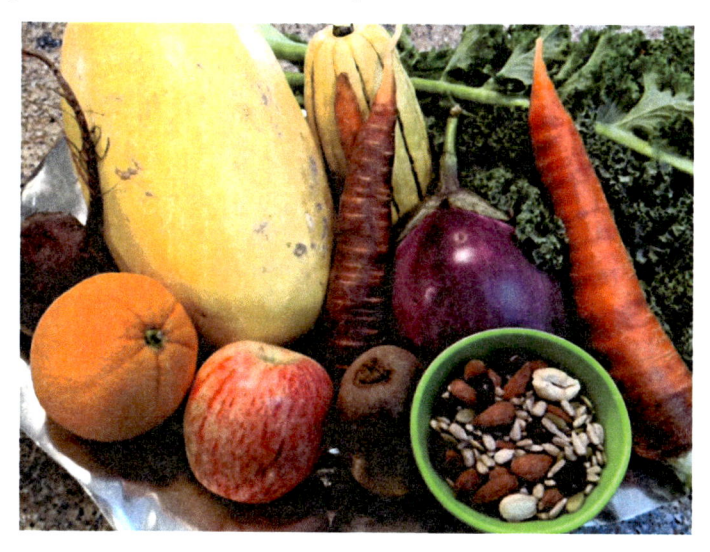

What Do the Colors On Your Plate Mean?
(*The Family Nutrition Book* by Dr. William Sears, MD and Martha Sears, RN)

Color:	Foods:	Nutrients/Benefit:
Yellow/Orange	Pumpkin, Sweet Potato Cantaloupe, Carrots, Apricots, Squash, Oranges	Vitamin A, Folic Acid, Beta Carotene, Fiber, Vitamin C *Improve skin, eyes, immune
Green	Broccoli, Leafy Greens (Spinach, Kale, Bok Choy) Brussel Sprouts, Cabbage	Vitamin A, Folic Acid, Calcium, carotenoids- *Antioxidants, immune. Sulforaphane- *Detoxify
Red	Strawberries, Tomato Raspberries, Red Pepper Watermelon, Apples, Beets	Lycopene, Vitamin C, Anthocyanins, *fight Cancer Antioxidant
Purple/Blue	Eggplant, Blueberries Grapes, Beets, Red Cabbage	Resveratrol, Phlavanoids Vitamin C, Antioxidants, *Boost Immune, fight cancer

If you feed your body junk, your body and mind will be junk. Feed your body healthy, whole foods not processed foods, and it will be healthy and strong. This is the lesson I teach my kids and the families I work with.

Foods higher in sugar are known to affect concentration and energy levels. High sugar and low fiber foods tend to spike your blood sugar which leads to a blood sugar crash, leaving the body feeling tired, lacking in focus, and feeling "ill" (dizzy, nauseous). It affects serotonin levels and mood as well.

So...I will say again, it is important to *balance* your foods, making healthy choices most of the time with an *occasional* not so healthy food if desired. The more good, healthy foods you eat, the less you want the not so healthy foods. It is referred to at the Institute for Integrative Nutrition as "crowding out." Fuel your body with plenty of fluid as well. These are guidelines on teaching kids about nutrition and healthy lifestyle choices. The reality is, kids know what is "good" for them, but they are also surrounded by hyper palatable foods that taste good. They fire up the pleasure center (dopamine response), and offset the healthy body balance. It happens to us all, and NO

ONE can make great choices all the time. The hope is to lay a foundation of knowledge and healthy habits that kids can have in their toolbox for life. This is for everyone to remember, both parent and child.

The Stop Light Diet Food Guide

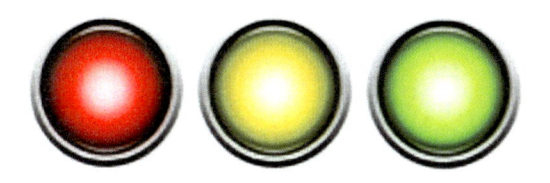

(Adapted from Epstein, L.H, Squirres, S. (1988) *The stoplight diet for children.* Boston: Little, Brown)

GREEN LIGHT FOODS: (GO)
Foods low in calories, high in nutrients.
- Eat as much as you need. (Green Drink = Water)
    - Whole fruit
    - Vegetables (plain, no butter, NOT corn, peas, potatoes)
    - Dried fruits and applesauce (no sugar added)

YELLOW LIGHT FOODS: (CAUTION)
Foods moderate in calories, high to moderate nutrients.
- Eat in moderation, can eat daily, but watch portions
  (Yellow Drink = Milk and seltzer or water with ¼ cup at most of juice)
    - Cheese and yogurt (dye free and no added sugar ideally) NOTE: *1 percent fat or more as they have less sugar, and studies are finding that the fat free versions are not as healthy as we once thought!*
    - Lean meats (turkey, chicken, pork, fish, low salt ham)
    - Eggs
    - Nuts and nut butters (one to two tablespoons)
    - Avocado, olives, olive oil, coconut oil, butter (grass fed), palm/sunflower/avocado oil
    - Whole grains (brown and wild rice, faro, bulgur, oats, amaranth, millet, quinoa, spelt, etc.)

- Hummus, cottage cheese, cream cheese, whole fruit jam or jelly
- Salad dressing (one teaspoon), homemade oil and vinegar is best
- Whole grain, high fiber crackers and granola bars (low sugar, mostly nut and grains. *Look out for hidden sugars such as cane, rice or other syrups, molasses, dates, agave nectar, or honey.)
- One to two ounces of dark Chocolate (made with 60 percent or more cacao)
- Coffee, teas, cocoa, wine (all unsweetened, and one to two cups max for caffeinated beverages, four to eight ounces of wine)

RED LIGHT FOODS: (STOP)
High calorie, high saturated or trans-fat, low nutrients.
- Eat occasionally, not daily or even weekly.
  (Red Drink = Soda, juice and juice drink/cocktail, sports drinks, powdered drinks, energy drinks, sweet teas)
  - Candy
  - Cookies
  - Cakes
  - Chips
  - Donuts, muffins (store bought)
  - Bagels
  - Ice cream
  - Pizza
  - Chicken Nuggets (not homemade)
  - Macaroni and cheese
  - Hot dogs
  - Pasta and breads
  - Snack crackers
  - Low fiber, high sugar granola bars and cereal bars
  - Red meat
  - Processed foods in general

Chapter 2

How to Get Your Family to Eat Healthier and Connect

Here are some ideas to expand your taste buds, get more vegetables in your diet (remember, we are supposed to get five to nine fruits and vegetables a day!), and keep your body and brain fueled well to perform well. If you just cannot get enough fruits and veggies in your diet, maybe try a dehydrated, encapsulated form, like Juice Plus (www.juiceplus.com). Eating the whole foods is preferred, as they contain everything your body needs to digest, balance, and absorb the nutrients into your system to maintain homeostasis.

- Create a food day of the week to help with variety, such as: "Meatless Monday," "Try it Tuesday" (and try new foods), "Whatever Wednesday" (eat leftovers), or "Kids Choice Friday" Be creative!

- Stay away from High Fructose Corn Syrup (HFCS) and extra sugars. Added sugars can actually upset your body's hormone regulating system and creates a sweeter "sweet tooth," especially HFCS. Try natural sweeteners like honey and pure maple syrup, but just a little. Limit sugar intake to less than twenty-five grams per day. Read labels for hidden sugars… (A 100 percent juice box has at least twenty-four grams of sugar!)

- Avoid anything with artificial color, flavor or scent. They are made from petroleum base! They have heavy metals that some people react strongly to. They are banned outside the US. There are links to ADHD, autism, hyperactivity, asthma, and tumors. For more information, go to: www.feingoldinstitute.org.

- Put veggies in your grains to increase your veggie intake. Add sautéed spinach, broccoli, or kale chopped in quinoa, faro, or rice. Diced or mashed squash, broccoli, or cauliflower can be put in pasta, rice, or risotto, even mac and cheese.

- Buy meats and fish that are locally raised and caught for better nutrition and to lower your "carbon footprint." Less travel time, and less processing involved. (For more information, visit www.localharvest.org or try the free "Seafood Watch" App from Monterey Bay Aquarium)

- Try to look for produce grown in USA and close to where you live. Go to Farmers' Markets or join a CSA (Community Shared Agriculture). Lots of produce comes from South America and Mexico in the late fall and winter. These areas have unclean water and minimal food regulations to follow. Kids are getting Hepatitis A shots because of ingesting produce from South America! Try buying local/seasonal and freezing for the winter or buying frozen organic grown in US.

Buy the following organic produce when you can: (Dirty Dozen)

Apples	Kale
Bell peppers	Lettuce
Carrots	Nectarine
Celery	Peach
Cherries	Pear
Grapes (if imported)	Strawberries

Plus: Eggs, Chicken, Turkey, Pork and Grass-fed Beef and Bison. *A new addition to this list is Green Beans.

Here's a general rule to follow: if it has a thick skin that you peel, you do not need to buy organic.

THE INFAMOUS GRAIN
Breaking Down the Pros and Cons.

There are many "diets" and research claims out there, be it from Paleo/Caveman proponents, Dr. David Perlmutter, author of *Grain Brain*, or Dr. William Davis, author of *Wheat Belly*, that tout grains as being "bad" or "silent killers" of the brain. There is lots of talk and cautions regarding Genetically Modified Organism (GMO). One of the main groups fighting for labeling GMO is the Environmental Working Group, supported by Dr. Mark Hyman, Founder and CEO of the Ultra Wellness Center in Lennox, MA.

Research from Harvard and the famous Nurses Study has shown the benefits of whole grains to cardiovascular health and to reducing inflammation, such as in Dr. Andrew Weil's Anti-Inflammatory Diet. In sifting through the various research, and even speaking with Dr. Perlmutter on my radio show, it seems that, as in most things, moderation and carefully chosen, minimally processed grains are the least likely to contribute to health issues. It is true that whole wheat and its products have contributed to some health challenges and symptoms such as fatigue, gastrointestinal upset, and even aches and pains from the gluten, a protein contained in wheat, rye, barley and bulgur. The problem lays in the "gluten free" fad, which has created another processed, high sugar product to hit the markets. Bottom line, again, is stick to whole grains, minimally processed, such as oats, brown and wild rice, spelt, amaranth, millet and quinoa. All are high in iron, protein, fiber, zinc and folic acid. Fiber helps clear the arteries and intestines and helps keep the body in balance.

Tips for Cooking for Kids:
- Let your kids help you choose, giving them a say in the menu.
- When introducing a new vegetable, make sure one they know and like is also on plate. For example, try grated beets or red cabbage on salad with carrots and cucumbers.
- Let kids help you cook in age appropriate ways—they will be more likely to try the food! Chop Chop Magazine is great for this. As previously mentioned, create food days of the week: "Meatless Monday," "New Food Friday," and "Breakfast for Dinner Wednesday."
- Eat as a family as much as possible. Turn OFF the TV, cell phones, and computers. MONKEY SEE, MONKEY DO, so pull, don't push in the right direction. You lead, and they will follow.

- Plan meals ahead based on the activities of the day. If we have activities in the evening, I plan a crock-pot meal. I have a white board on my fridge with the week's meals planned out, so the kids know what's for dinner, and I am not trying to plan at the witching hour just before dinner.

I want to add a side note regarding kids and teaching them to make healthy choices. I am of the practical mindset that the goal is not to "control" our kids' food choices, but to teach them how to make good, healthy choices, listen to their body and mindfully eat. I would love to say that my kids always make healthy choices, but that is not the reality nor is it practical. Peer pressure, and the targeted derailing by the food industry making the "bad" foods taste so good, can cause kids to binge, crave sweets/fat and make some not so great choices, particularly in adolescents. If there is a pan of brownies in front of me, I can try my best to resist, but chances are, I will eat one, or two or three... The point is, the more "controlling" we are as parents, oftentimes, the more our kids may binge, hide food, and mindlessly eat. The key is getting as much healthy whole food in them when you can and creating an environment conducive to this at home.

In addition, if you decide, as an adult, to try a specific kind of diet, be it vegetarian, vegan, paleo, I caution you not to make your kids or family follow it right off the bat. Try it out yourself first, and then decide if you want to have your family follow that path. Everyone has their own unique needs as far as what foods work for them based on energy levels, development, and biochemical make up, and what works for one person may not work for others. It is called bio-individuality, a term I picked up from Joshua Rosenthal, founder of The Institute for Integrative Nutrition.

Aim for a healthy, whole food, mostly plant-based diet with meat and/or grains on the side as options. Listen to your body, pay attention to your energy, your skin, and bowel movements. It tells you a lot about how the gut is working to digest the food. Your body will stay healthy and function well if you fuel it with the right fuel.

Based on the research from Harvard School of Public Health, Mayo Clinic, T. Colin Campbell's China Study, the Harvard Nurses Study, the Framingham Heart Study, and recent research findings published in top medical journals such as the New England Journal of Medicine and The American Journal of Clinical Nutrition, the following *GENERAL* dietary guidelines can be made, obviously, as stated above, fine tuning based on your individual and your children's individual needs.

1. Eat a mostly whole food, plant based diet rich in a variety of vegetables, nuts, seeds, and legumes.

2. Eat plenty of healthy, minimally processed fats such as olive oil, coconut oil, avocado, olives and nuts, and lean proteins based on your body's needs, be it from plant or animal. ***Modified Mediterranean or Paleo-Vegan Diet.**

3. Avoid added sugar—especially processed foods. (It is closely linked to inflammation and cancer.)

4. Use sea salt and iodine rich foods, like seaweed, seafood, cranberries, poultry/dairy, navy and lima beans, spinach, Swiss chard, garlic, and strawberries. Iodine supports the thyroid and metabolism. *Did you know that most of the salt we ingest is iodized salt containing low iodine? Seventy percent of our salt intake comes from processed foods that are low in iodine...*

5. Drink water—lots of it! Minimize the juice, even 100 percent fruit juice as it affects the body homeostasis and blood sugar like sugar, and soft drinks causing spikes and insulin surges leading to excess fat storage.

6. Eat whole, minimally processed grains, mainly gluten free, such as quinoa, brown and wild rice, millet, buckwheat, and oats. Avoid excess bread, pasta and cereal, as processed food.

7. Plan ahead for meals and snacks, as being prepared stops impulsive hunger binges and keeps you eating mindfully. Cut up vegetables, hard boil eggs, and plan out menus for the week around your week's activities. I map it out on a white board on my fridge!

WHAT TO STOCK IN YOUR KITCHEN

Fruits and Vegetables:
- Carrots
- Zucchini
- Cucumber
- Leeks
- Shallots and garlic
- Red and yellow onion
- Celery
- Spinach (fresh & frozen)
- Kale
- Scallion/green onion
- Squash (acorn, butternut, delicate)
- Colored peppers
- Broccoli
- Green beans (fresh or frozen)
- Lemon
- Potatoes (sweet and new)
- Cabbage – Napa, red, green
- Beets
- Lettuce and Greens

Grains and Flours:
- Brown Rice
- Barley
- Mixed Grain (spelt/rice/barley/millet)
- Whole grain pasta
- Faro
- Rice Noodles/Soba (buckwheat) noodles
- Wheat berries
- Panko bread crumbs
- Dry and canned beans (black white cannellini, red kidney, lentil, chickpeas)
- Whole wheat pastry flour, spelt flour, almond flour
- Corn meal/polenta
- Oats, (organic) and oat flour
- Flax seed (ground or whole)

Spices and Condiments:
- Grainy Dijon mustard
- Good quality local honey
- Organic, low sodium chicken and vegetable stock
- Tube of tomato paste
- Good quality organic salsa
- Low sodium soy sauce
- Variety of vinegars: balsamic, rice wine, red wine, white distilled, and cider
- Pure Maple Syrup
- Good quality Vanilla extract
- EVOO (Extra Virgin Olive Oil) and cooking spray
- Coconut oil
- Toasted sesame oil
- SPICES: sage, thyme, curry, rosemary, fennel, cumin, chili, nutmeg, cinnamon, ginger, basil, oregano, sea salt, pepper
- White Miso Paste

Protein and Meats (Ideally Organic):
- Pork tenderloin or loin
- Rotisserie chicken
- Chicken cutlets/thighs
- Pancetta/Prosciutto
- Ground turkey chicken
- Eggs
- Goat Cheese and Feta
- Parmesan/grated cheese
- Edemame (FROZEN)
- Tofu-firm and silk
- Beans and lentils
- Nuts: Peanuts, pine, pecan, almonds, walnuts, cashews
- Nut butters
- Kefir, cultured milk
- Coconut or almond milk
- Yogurt – plain and Greek

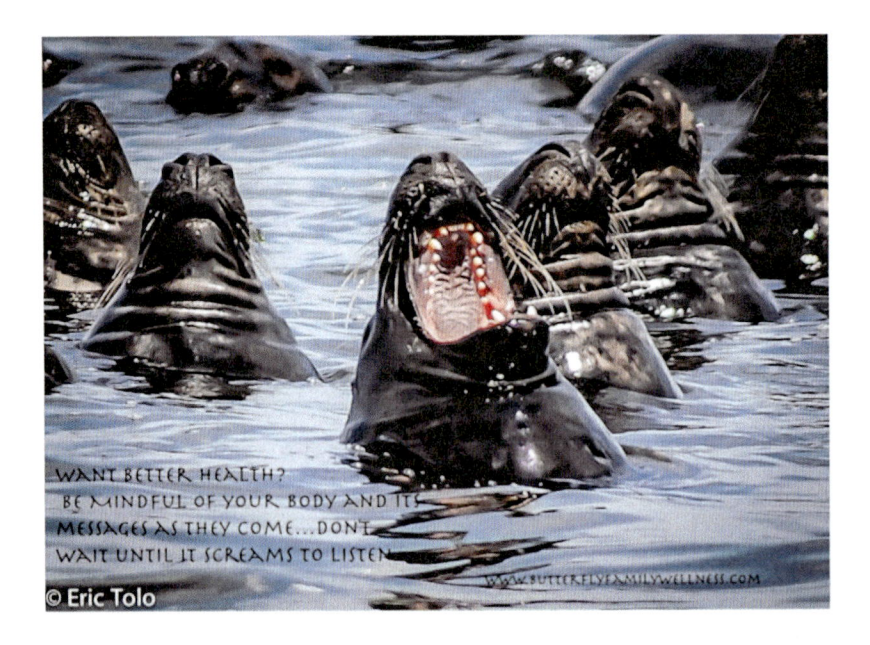

TOP 7 THINGS TO INCORPORATE IN YOUR FAMILY DIET:

1) **Healthy Fats**: Olive oil, avocado, olives, coconut oil nuts (especially walnuts and almonds). These have Omega 3 Fatty acids, which help with brain function, memory and help lubricate joints and build neurotransmitters to aid with the body's balance.
2) **Cruciferous Vegetables**: Broccoli, cabbage, Brussel sprouts. These contain sulforaphane, which helps the body to fight and purge toxins.
3) **Green Leafy Vegetables**: Kale, spinach, Swiss chard, darker lettuce. These contain high amounts of calcium and B vitamins like Folate. They help the body detoxify and regenerate cells.
4) **Berries**: Blueberries, strawberries, raspberries, cranberry, goji berries, acai berries. These are strong antioxidants with the Vitamin C and Flavanoids. These tasty beauties help with inflammation, circulation and regeneration of cells.
5) **Fish**: Healthy, sustainable shellfish, Alaskan cod, wild salmon, haddock and smaller bait fish like sardines, anchovies, and herring. They have healthy Omega 3 fatty acid and help with memory, cognitive function neurotransmitters, and cell/body lubrication for joint, skin, and eye

health.
6) **Apples and beets** for their cleansing properties and antioxidant benefit.
7) **Natural Probiotic**: Sauerkraut, yogurt, and kimchi (fermented cabbage) for their gut health benefits.

Strive for variety of food and color. Each color in veggies and fruits give different nutrient and mineral. Eat the WHOLE fruits or veggies versus juicing, as the whole fruit has everything the body needs to digest and absorb all of the nutrients and slow down digestion, like fiber.

TOP CONVERSATION STARTERS TO CONNECT AT FAMILY MEALTIME

Sitting together as a family at a meal is the best way to stay connected as a family, slow down and be present with your food, self, and the people you love. Create "Rules and Expectations" around meal time to foster healthy habits: no reading, electronics, TV at the family meal; no work during family meal, and stay seated until everyone is done, so people do not rush. I have even created a "Family Fuel Placemat" with a child client to remind the family to slow down, engage with each other, and be present in the moment, without judgment. Here are some ideas to start the conversation and connection.

1. What was the best part of your day? Go around to each person. Or, what was a high of the day?
2. Did you do anything, see anything, or have anything done that was nice or inspiring?
3. What was the challenge for the day?
4. What did you learn today? (Every day brings opportunity for growth and learning. It is when we are closed minded to lessons that we stop growing and evolving.)
5. What made you laugh or smile today?
6. What are you grateful for today? (This can be a tough one for kids, but we can teach by example.)

The key is to just allow conversation to flow, without judgment, and practicing good listening and responding versus reacting. When kids feel heard and truly listened to without judgment, it is one of the best gifts of connection and unconditional love you can give them. If you do not know how, or find yourself reacting or judging, the first step is awareness, and with that, you can seek the help and tools to change. That is a great lesson to kids as well!

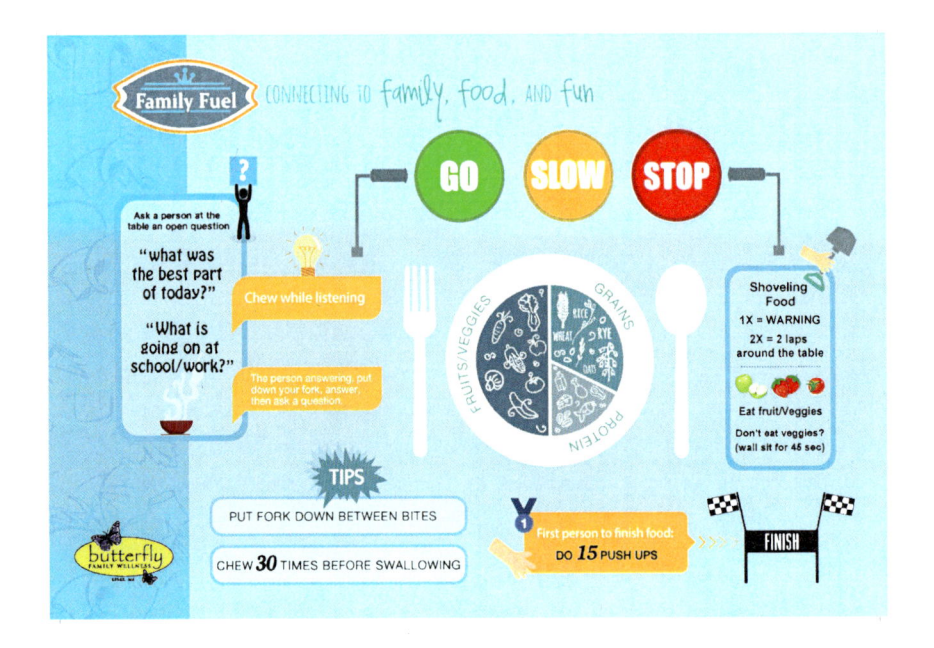

Family Fuel — CONNECTING TO family, food, AND fun

Ask a person at the table an open question

"what was the best part of today?"

"What is going on at school/work?"

Chew while listening

The person answering, put down your fork, answer, then ask a question.

GO   SLOW   STOP

FRUITS/VEGGIES   GRAINS   PROTEIN

Shoveling Food
1X = WARNING
2X = 2 laps around the table

Eat fruit/Veggies
Don't eat veggies? (wall sit for 45 sec)

TIPS
PUT FORK DOWN BETWEEN BITES
CHEW 30 TIMES BEFORE SWALLOWING

First person to finish food: DO 15 PUSH UPS

FINISH

butterfly FAMILY WELLNESS

Chapter 3

Recipe for Whole Health and Wellness

2 cups of mindfulness: an awareness of self at present moment without judgment. It helps relieve stress and anxiety, creates awareness of self and surroundings, and has been shown to alleviate stress, boost immune system, and reduce inflammatory process. It has been said that anxiety is future focused while depression is focused on the past. Be in the moment of today.

1/2 cup of quiet: A moment of stillness to check in with self and others, so you can listen to the messages. Be present and still in the moment, so you can be open to receive information and connect.

1 cup of good listening: Many of us react, interrupt, or get distracted when someone speaks to us. If we are present, quiet, and open, we can listen and respond in a thoughtful way. (It is tough but essential for good communication.) If you do not have this tool in your toolbox, seek help to get this tool and practice.

2 cups of communication: This is vital to healthy relationships, healthy emotions, and energy flow through the body. It opens the throat chakra and allows feelings, desires, and needs be heard. Again, this can be tricky, but if you do not have this tool, there are people and professionals who can help you get it! In my opinion, relationships break down between couples, parents and children, and friends when communication breaks down. Poor communication is a breeding ground for resentment, frustration, and disconnect.

2-3 cups of whole food: This is the fuel for your body and brain. For body balance and stability, stick to real, unprocessed foods—mostly lean proteins, fruits and veggies, and whole grains. Minimize sugar and processed foods.

1 cup of exercise: Make time to move, and sometimes, get breathless. Move your body for thirty to sixty minutes, fifteen to twenty of which your heart rate is 85 percent heart rate max. Mix up the cardiovascular and weight bearing exercises to boost metabolism and strengthen bones and connective tissue. Avoid prolonged periods of being sedentary; take movement breaks for the brain and to prevent inflammation. Go to CDC.org for guidelines on exercise for different ages.

1 cup of connection: Take time, create time, to spend with people who matter in your life. Studies show people who connect with others lead longer, healthier lives. "Time is a created thing. To say 'I don't have time' is like saying 'I don't want to do it'." - Cheryl Richardson

Dash of chaos: It is good for endorphins, perspective, and health to have a bit of chaos. It creates sharper reactions and problem solving skills and keeps body system alive and on point. One of my favorite quotes is, "Peace. It does not mean to be in a place where there is no noise, trouble, or hard work. It means to be in the midst of those things and still be calm in your heart."- unknown.

1 cup of play and laughter: It is believed to boost the immune system and relieve stress, and it helps people connect. It is very freeing to let go and not take yourself so seriously. I find my family connects best this way, through play. My kids love when my husband and I play soccer, football, or just bounce on the trampoline with them. We even had a lip-sync contest for my birthday! My sixteen-year-old won. It was hilarious. They laugh at us (with us), but we laugh at ourselves!

When I hear of someone going through an illness, or an illness of a child, my advice to people who want to help is to help them remember to laugh. That is what I needed when my son was sick. Not to always talk about it but to escape, momentarily, through play and laugh.

1 cup self-care (or time doing what you truly enjoy): It fills your energy well that others may drink from. On the airplane, the flight attendant reminds parents to put their oxygen mask on first before putting on their child's. Why? Because, if you pass out or get sick or run down, how can you help or be there for your kids? Taking time for yourself is a great example to set for your kids. It is a reminder that you are important too.

Most clients that come to me, especially moms, are so busy running around and doing for everyone else that their own physical and emotional health gets neglected. I find I am more present and patient with my family when I have taken a bit of time for myself, be it a run, yoga, or even a hot bath...alone!

1/2 cup of gratitude: Being grateful helps us be present in the moment and appreciate what we have versus don't have. It helps create perspective. Society is often highlighting what we do not have or what else we "need" to be happy. Happiness comes from within, not from external things. Practicing daily gratitude by writing or stating what you are grateful for today is a great way to reflect and find inner peace.

1/2 cup of slow deep breaths: Slow, purposeful breathing has been shown to activate the relaxation response and counters cortisol release. It helps stabilize hormones and slows the "fight or flight" response we often get with stress.

1 cup of moderation: Go ahead, eat, drink, play, work.... find your balance. Do not over-indulge, or deprive, but moderate. Extremes either way, be it deprivation or indulgence, often bring the body out of balance.

2 cups of good quality sleep (six to eight hours minimum): The body releases cytokines, our anti-inflammatory messengers, in our deepest phase of sleep. It is our body's healing and regenerating period. Studies have shown that chronic bouts of less than six to seven hours of sleep affects our focus and exposes our bodies to prolonged cortisol release—the body stress hormone, which can lead to inflammation and disease.

1 cup of kindness: Practice acts of kindness. It is contagious and brings more happiness than doing for oneself. It ripples compassion and helps spread good cheer and feelings of wellbeing.

Sporadic bouts of letting go: Let go of perfection, release control, and just ride the roller coaster of life. There are times when trying to control something just creates stress and resentment, and impedes connections. You can control you—and your reactions/responses—but no one else's. Work on responding versus reacting, which comes from listening, stepping back, taking deep breaths, and being mindful. Letting go can be stressful for some people who need to be in control of their environment. However, learning to let go, even just a little, can be freeing and empowering. Life is full of uncertainties. Once we trust that we have the tools needed to handle whatever life throws our way, we can let go and be free to enjoy our life.

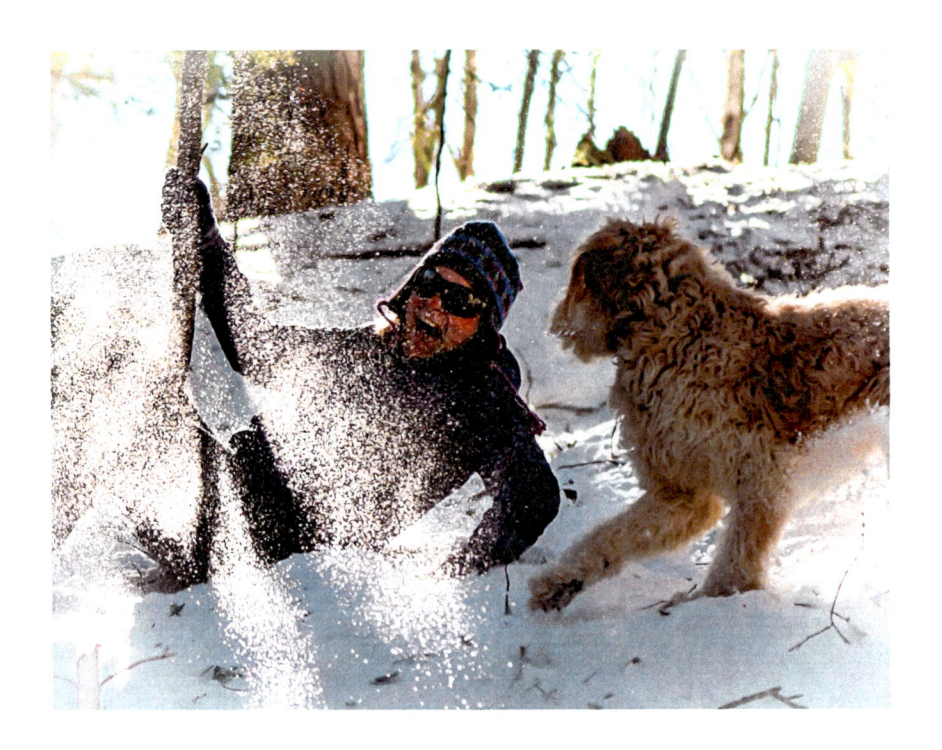

Chapter 4

Tips for Creating Healthy Habits for Your Family

One of the most important things to remember is that your actions, habits, and awareness truly impact the habits and actions of your children. Being aware of some habits that do not serve you and seeking change is a very powerful message for kids to see. Kids are so much more observant and aware than we tend to give them credit for. This generation of kids in particular tends to be very aware of incongruity of messages, hypocrisy, as well as someone trying to pull one over on them. It amazes me that they are able to be duped by the food industry, as they are reeling kids into an addiction to sugar, fat, and "quick on the go" food habits. These messages, as well as the messages on television programs geared towards children, can be very misleading, and very derailing to healthy habits, healthy connections, and respectful and open communication. Not only is it important to be aware of our own actions, choices, and environment, but it is essential that we are tapped in and aware of what is going on in our children's world—namely their environment, exposures, and integrated messages. One of the greatest gifts and greatest investments into your child's future health is the gift of time, connection, and awareness.

Be present in your life and your child's life. We all can get caught up and busy with our own "stuff," but acknowledging when this occurs, be it from the feeling of being disconnected, short fused, or unaware, it is never too late to stop, slow down, and connect. When we, as parents, are aware and accountable, we teach our children to be. As I tell my kids and myself on a daily basis, OWN YOUR ACTIONS.

Here are a few tips on how to connect and create healthy habits:

- Unplug from phones, electronics, and TV. Create a time and space that is unplugged, such as dinner or meals. This leads to conversation, connection, and stillness, which facilitates awareness and accountability. If you, as a parent, are always plugged in, the message that sends is that you do not want to take the time to connect. Telling kids to unplug when we do not screams hypocrisy. This is a wedge between connecting, especially to tweens and teens.

- Create time to DO something together as a family or one on one. This does not need to be daily, but weekly, every few weeks, or once a month. Teens and tweens will balk at this, but if you get their input—give them options—they will secretly or outwardly enjoy time you give them. Here is the key: make it fun and embrace your inner play. As embarrassed as kids can be with parents acting goofy, when we can laugh, joke, and be playful, that truly helps us connect to our kids. Here are some ideas: Go for a hike, bike ride, or walk; bounce on the trampoline; play tag or manhunt. Play a game, be it sports, a board game, or even a video game. DO NOT GET TOO COMPETITIVE OR CRITICAL as that can derail the whole connecting process. You choose what you enjoy and what kids enjoy and get on their level. It makes them feel heard and important.

- If you do not eat well and eat healthy, do not expect your kids to. Work together to create a healthy food environment. If your child needs to lose weight, DO NOT make it about them. Make it about being healthy as a family. At the same time, if you are constantly dieting or depriving, that can create body image issues in your children. We can all stand to make some healthy changes, so offer support, not criticism. We are all a part of the problem as well as the solution.

- Move your body daily. When you show that exercise and moving versus sedentary behavior is important to you, you show your kids that it is important. Studies have shown that too much sitting or sedentary behavior is linked to inflammation and chronic disease. It is suggested that we move our bodies every twenty minutes to decrease the effects of inactivity on our body health. For exercise guidelines, check out www.cdc.org/physicalactivity/everyone/. If you are exercising with your children, make sure it is age appropriate and not adult exercise for kids. Small children and school age kids are interval exercisers, meaning they have short bursts of energy followed by recovery periods. Tweens and teens can exercise longer and a bit more intensely, but in order to create a healthy habit of movement and exercise, the activity needs to be fun, engaging, and appealing. So check in with them, and find something to do together.

- Choose your words carefully. Positive words to self and to others bring positive energy and are uplifting, so you can soar. Negative words and overly critical comments can weigh people down like a rock and create discouragement, leading to low self-esteem and negative behaviors. I often tell clients who are negative to self or to kids, to have two jars or bowls visible. I tell them to collect rocks and feathers. When they catch themselves, or their kids point out the negative words, place a rock in a jar. If you can change the negative to positive, or say something positive and encouraging, you place a feather in the other jar. This creates a visual and helps with accountability and awareness. Bringing kids or a spouse into the exercise, asking for support, is a great way to connect and creates an atmosphere of positivity and accountability.

- Work on your perspective. Save your arguments and need for control for things that are truly important to you and your children's well-being. When we learn to let go a bit and release the unattainable concept of perfection, we can start to appreciate the little things in life and appreciate each other. Now, this is coming from a total type A person who has worked very hard at this with much (but not total) success. My mantras, two I repeat to myself and my kids often are:

1) You can control you and your actions and how you respond to others, but you cannot control anyone else.
2) Take back your power, and do not give it away. If you are responsible for something, own it. If not and you are just reacting then let it go, saying "that is not mine, that is yours."

This is a journey, not a race, but practicing these mantras, sharing them, and even sharing your struggle to embrace this with your kids, is a wonderful way to connect and create healthy habits together, leading by example.

- Finally, as much as we want to pave the way and smooth out the road for our kids, it is the experience of overcoming the bumps in the road and the lessons gained from these experiences that give them tools for their toolbox of life. Trust me, I know how hard it is to watch your child struggle and get knocked down by life, but it is so uplifting and rewarding to all when they feel supported and empowered to get back up, dust themselves off, and keep moving forward on their path. Help your child fill up their toolbox. Offer support, but as long as its age appropriate, do not take over. Instead, let them explore and experience the world around them.

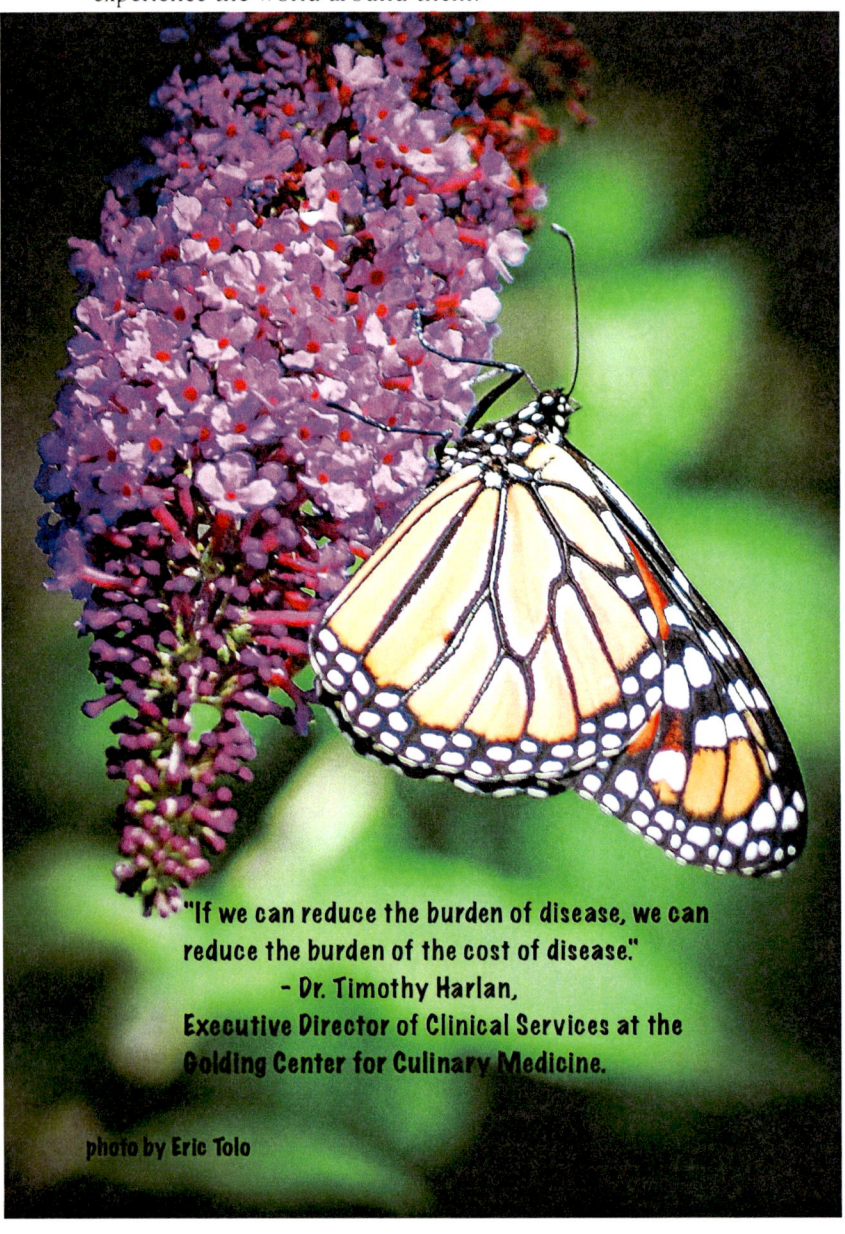

"If we can reduce the burden of disease, we can reduce the burden of the cost of disease."
- Dr. Timothy Harlan,
Executive Director of Clinical Services at the Golding Center for Culinary Medicine.

photo by Eric Tolo

Chapter 5

Elimination Plan: Figuring Out What You May Be Sensitive To

Many of us have tried to lose weight or body fat, or fluctuate with how our clothes fit. Some of us have allergies, skin irritation, asthma, GI upset, or autoimmune problems that food can often exacerbate. We need to tap into what we are eating and see how we react to certain foods and to our environment. We sometimes need to cleanse our body of the many toxins stored in our liver, "reboot" our bodies to function, cleanse, and heal as it was meant to. In doing this we can rid ourselves of the cravings and bad habits we tend to lapse into, which keep us in this vicious cycle. We can also avoid inflammatory flair ups that can lead to illness or discomfort.

I run a Mindful Eating Reset "Cleanse," which is NOT a fast and does not have "forbidden" foods. It starts out with a restricted elimination diet for two weeks, followed by a slow introduction of "reactive" foods. The focus is on eating closer to the earth and on being more mindful of the quality, content, sustainability, and environmental impact of what we choose to eat and surround our self with.

I recommend keeping a food journal daily for the four weeks. In the journal you can note: how you feel when waking, when eating, and at the end of the day, paying close attention to energy, hunger, stress, and bowel patterns and consistency. All of these things will help with understanding your body and mind, your triggers and pitfalls, as well as how your body is responding to toxins, ridding itself of toxins, and the impact of specific foods.

Many adults have issues resulting from the body's clearing house or cleaners, the kidney and the liver, which can become overworked and sluggish. There are naturopaths and holistic health practitioners out there that offer liver and kidney cleanse, or supplements, to detoxify the body. I am a believer of gentle resets for the system through whole foods, elimination diets, and lots of water to flush out the system.

I usually start with figuring out what a person could be exposed to that is creating "DIS-ease" in the body. Some integrative practitioners use something called "muscle testing." This is where one holds a food or a product they question. The practitioner then has them hold out their arms and resist as they push down on the arm. The premise is that you will be able to resist with your muscles engaged when the product is beneficial to you. If you react to the product, then your muscles have trouble resisting and the arm is pushed down easily. For me, this system does not work clearly. I am too stubborn and tend to "muscle it." I am then not clear of the result.

I prefer to use a pendulum, and test products by dowsing. Dowsing can be done by anyone and gives a clear "yes" or "no." I hold the pendulum up and down, asking to be shown my "yes" or "no." For me, my yes is a circle motion, and my no is a swing up and back. I then ask a clear closed question like, "Is this bread good for me?" The pendulum swings either in a circular motion or up and back telling me the answer. You really have to try it to believe it. It is actually pretty cool and something that connects you to your own inner knowing or intuition. We often have a sense when something is not working for us.

The elimination diet is a way to rule out food items that we are concerned we may be reacting to. The most common food items people are sensitive to are: gluten or wheat products, dairy, peanuts and tree nuts, sugar, and with some sensitive individuals—salicylates. Salicylates are chemicals found naturally in some plants and sometimes added to some products, like aspirin or beauty products, lotions, and soaps. For a list of salicylates, go to www.webmd.com/allergies/guide/salicylate-allergy. Some of these food items are apples, oranges, some cruciferous vegetables, stone fruits, and berries to name a few.

There are varying degrees of salicylate sensitivities or allergies. I recommend working with a specialist to help sift through the complicated realm of severe allergies and food sensitivities.

For people wondering what is contributing to abdominal or gastrointestinal discomfort, fatigue, or even joint aches, the following basic elimination diet can help guide you to your body's messages and mindful eating.

THE ELIMINATION PLAN:
Weeks 1-2
Figure out what your body is "reactive" to by starting a two-week elimination diet. This will also help with ridding your bodies of toxins and cravings. It

begins with **avoiding eating/drinking:** dairy (cow), wheat and gluten, refined sugar, artificial sweeteners, red meat (beef, lamb and pork), and alcohol. The plan is to **eat closer to the earth, minimally processed foods, drink two or more cups of green tea and lots of water, and eat lots of green leafy veggies and lean protein.** This is to help liver function, rid the body of toxins, and boost the body's ability to burn fat and burn energy efficiently. The goal is to decrease body fat, decrease cravings, and increase energy and alertness.

Drink lots of water—starting the day with a glass of room temperature water first thing in the morning. Keep a journal to record what you eat, how you feel, and what your energy and bowl habits are. Some people will feel ill with headaches, nausea, and irritability. This is often the toxins coming out, and the body trying to balance itself. It usually only lasts for the first few days.

Weeks 3-4
You can add in goat cheese and plain Greek yogurt (you can add honey). You can slowly add in harder cheeses, used in moderation, but see how you feel. I recommend avoiding drinking milk, cow's milk at this point as that is the hardest for our body to process. After a week, add in dairy and see how you feel; you can add in wheat products, but do so sparingly and with caution. This is one of the biggest contributors to women and weight gain and fluctuation, as well as autoimmune and inflammatory flair ups.

Again, pay attention to how you feel and to cravings. Start out with sprouted grains and whole grains, continuing to avoid pasta, refined grains, and breads. It is vital you pay attention to how you feel and don't "cheat" during the elimination part, as you will not really reset your system and will not truly see if that food item is a sensitive one for you. Another caution is to make sure you pick a time to do this where you are not traveling, eating out, or at friends' and relatives' homes. You really need to plan and commit to this journey if you are seeking information about your body and health.

If, at the end of this mini elimination, you remain not feeling well or with unanswered questions, I recommend seeing a holistic health coach, naturopath (with caution, as they can be very expensive and extreme with recommendations), or a registered dietician with an integrative approach. Sadly, many doctors are not versed in nutrition and the effects of foods on the body's systems.

One last caution: be careful of severe or extreme and overly restrictive plans. There is a time and a place for extremes, and often, an extreme plan can lead to offsetting the body's balance system even more. Overly restrictive diets, especially for normally cognitive functioning kids, are difficult to stick with long term. What works for one person, in general, does not always translate to working for you. It is important to find out what works or does not work for you, the individual. I know I have mentioned this earlier, but... I feel it is a crucial point. Feel free to play, explore different dietary options. I am here to support you on your path to health.

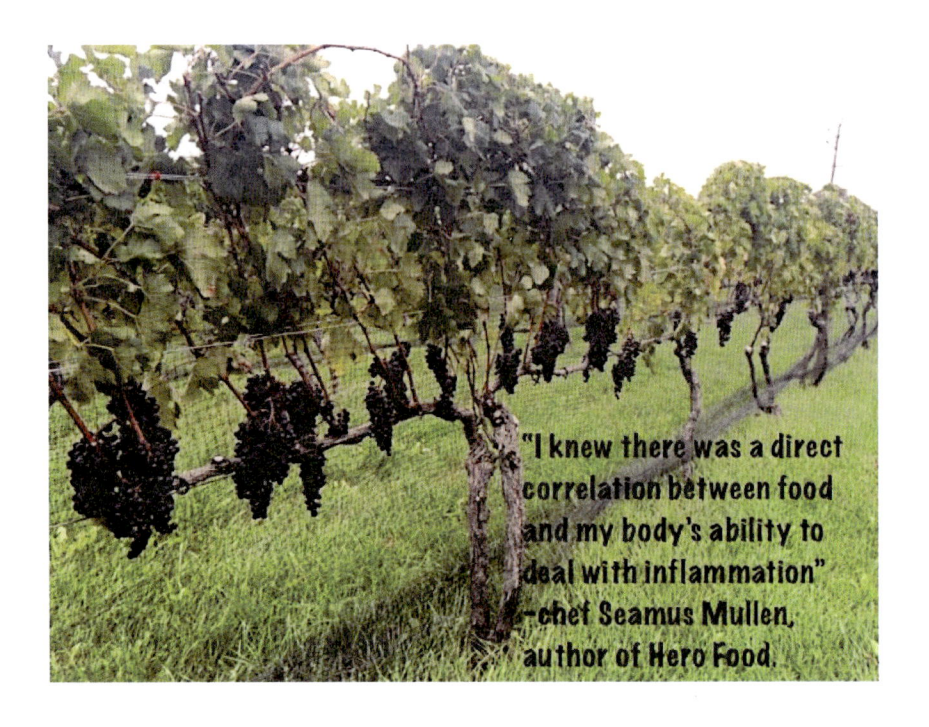

"I knew there was a direct correlation between food and my body's ability to deal with inflammation"
-chef Seamus Mullen, author of Hero Food.

Chapter 6

Morning Fuel: Breakfast

"One cannot think well, love well, sleep well if one has not dined well"- Virginia Woolf

Oh My Oatmeal
1-2 cups of quick cook oats	*NOTE: ½ cup per person*
2-4 cups of milk of choice	*NOTE: 1 cup per person*
2-4 tablespoons chopped walnuts
2-4 teaspoons maple syrup
½ cups fresh or frozen berries per serving

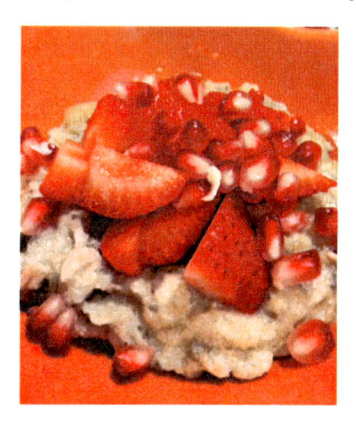

Heat milk in sauce pan, bringing to a gentle boil. Add oats and cook to thicken. Once liquid is mostly absorbed, add walnuts, maple syrup, and blueberries. Remove from heat, mix to combine, and serve.

• • •

Protein Power Pancakes with Blueberry Compote (makes 4-6 pancakes)
½ cup whole oats
½ banana
2 tablespoons plain Greek yogurt or silken tofu (if dairy free)
1 teaspoon vanilla extract
1 egg
2 tablespoons walnuts

Mix in blender or Nutribullet. Pour onto heated, sprayed griddle into 2 inch rounds.

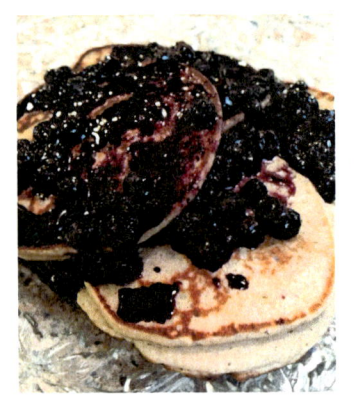

Blueberry Compote Topping:
Combine 1 cup frozen or fresh organic blueberries with 1-2 tablespoons of pure maple syrup. Heat over medium-low heat. Pour over pancakes.

WOW Waffles (makes 6-8 waffles)
1 ½ cups whole wheat, spelt, or oat flour
2 tablespoons wheat germ or ground flaxseeds (Omega 3)
2 teaspoons maple syrup
1 ½ teaspoons baking powder
½ teaspoon sea salt
1 ½ cups milk of choice
¼ cup safflower or sunflower oil
1 egg
1 teaspoon vanilla extract

Mix batter and pour into heated, greased waffle iron. Cook each for around one minute.

Top with sliced strawberries, blueberries, or raspberries and pure maple syrup or above compote.

Note: Spelt, although not gluten free, is high in zinc and less "reactive" or genetically modified than wheat. Oat flour can be GF, especially if you grind your own oats.

Poached Eggs with Kale and Shallot Sautee (serves 1-4)
2 eggs per person at room temperature
1-2 shallots, diced
1-4 cups of kale, shredded
1 teaspoon olive oil
2 teaspoons balsamic vinegar
Optional: 1 cup shitake mushrooms and/or tomatoes diced.

Boil water in a medium sauce pan. Add 1 teaspoon balsamic to water. As water starts to boil, begin to sauté shallots in olive oil. Add kale and any other vegetables to sauté. Add 1 teaspoon balsamic to pan when vegetables begin to soften. Toss and place in shallow bowl. Place eggs in a small cup, then slowly add eggs to boiling water using a slotted spoon to contain them. Cook for one to two minutes, depending on how runny you like them. Scoop eggs out with slotted spoon and place over sautéed vegetables.

NOTE: If poaching eggs is overwhelming, or not your thing, try to soft boil and place over veggies. If it's still not your thing, fry two eggs over easy and place on top of veggies. You can serve over an English muffin or sprouted grain toast as well.

. . .

Quick Quiche or Frittata
1 pie crust, store bought or home made
1 onion, diced
1 leek, sliced (just the white part)
1 glove garlic, minced
1 cup mushrooms (shitake, baby bellas)
1-2 cups spinach, Swiss chard, kale or broccoli, chopped
8 eggs
1 cup milk of choice
1 cup goat or cheddar, feta or Swiss cheese, crumbled or shredded (or mix of several cheeses)
1 teaspoon dry mustard
Salt and pepper
1 teaspoon thyme

1 teaspoon oregano
1-2 tomatoes chopped (optional)

Place pie crust or arrange sliced potato on bottom of pie plate. If using pie crust, press up along edge of plate and poke holes along bottom and edges with fork. Bake at 400 degrees for eight to ten minutes to slightly brown. Sauté onion, garlic, and leeks in olive oil. Add mushrooms and greens, and cook until softened. Remove from heat. In medium bowl, beat eggs and add milk, mustard seed, and cheese. Mix well. Add sautéed vegetables to egg mixture. Add salt, pepper, thyme, and oregano. Mix and pour into pie crust/ potato crust. Bake at 375 degrees for 30-35 minutes until top of quiche is firm.

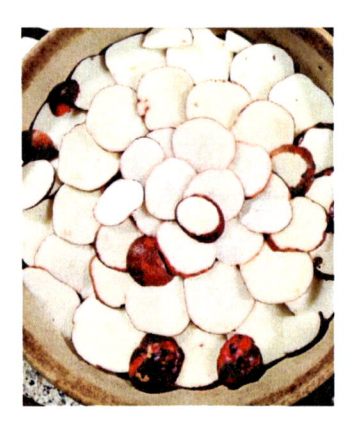

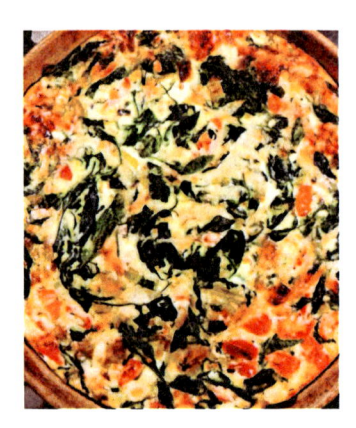

These can be done as without crust as well. For gluten free, use sweet or white potatoes as crust. Slice thin, arrange on bottom of pan or muffin tins, spray with olive oil, sprinkle with sea salt, and bake for ten minutes. Great breakfast to go!

Simple Solutions: (Quick, no fuss options)
Spread nut butter on a rice cake or sprouted grain toast with sliced banana or strawberries.

Yogurt (plain Greek or low sugar vanilla) with berries & almonds or granola.

Chapter 7

Soups, Salad and Vegetable

"Soup is a lot like a family. Each ingredient enhances the others; each batch has its own characteristics; and it needs time to simmer to reach full flavor." - Marge Kennedy

Squash Apple Soup

1 butternut squash peeled, seeded and cubed
1 tablespoon olive oil
1-2 shallots diced
1 granny smith apple or Fiji apple, peeled and diced
2-3 cups vegetable broth
1 teaspoon thyme
½ teaspoon salt
½ teaspoon pepper
1 tablespoon plain Greek yogurt or 1 tablespoon butter (if you like it a bit creamy)

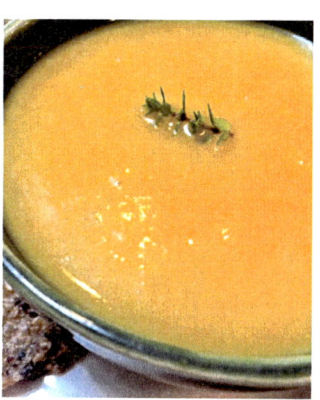

Sauté squash and shallots in olive oil until squash starts to soften. Add apples, and sauté until fragrant. Add broth, thyme, salt and pepper. Bring to boil. With a wand/stick blender, blend and purée soup mixture to smooth consistency. Add yogurt at the end and blend to mix. If soup is too thick, add more broth.

• • •

Miso Noodle Soup

½ cup white miso paste
4 cups of warm water
6 scallions, diced

4 ounces firm tofu, sliced into ½ inch cubes
¼ cup seaweed flakes or kelp
2-3 cups either spinach or bok choy, chopped
2 cups noodles of choice (soba, udon, Japanese curly or kelp noodles)

Mix miso paste and warm water in Dutch oven or soup pot. Stir to dissolve paste. Heat on medium to medium-low heat. Add scallions, tofu, sea vegetables and greens. Bring to a boil. Add the noodles and cook for 10 minutes. Serve in deep bowls.

Note: Sea vegetables contain Omega 3 and iodine, both things the body needs. Tofu is fermented soy, so it contains less phytoestrogen. You can substitute chicken though.

• • •

Fresh Tomato Basil Soup
4-5 ripe or overripe tomatoes, stems removed, rinsed, and cored.
1-2 shallots
1-2 cloves garlic
1 teaspoon sea salt
1 roasted red pepper (roast in oven at 400 degrees for ten to fifteen minutes)
½ cup fresh basil
¼ cup cashews or ¼ cup parmesan cheese (adds creaminess)

Sauté shallots and garlic in 1 teaspoon olive oil. Remove from heat. In Nutribullet, Vita mixer, or food processor, add tomatoes, basil, red pepper, and shallot/garlic mix. Add salt and ¾ of cashews or cheese, and blend until smooth and liquid. Pour into a sauce pan and heat. Serve warm and top with remaining cashews or parmesan cheese. My kids love this with grilled cheese!

• • •

Foundation Creation Soup
(Soup base with options to add in based on your mood and what is available)
1 large onion diced
2 cloves garlic
1 large leek, whites halved and sliced
2 carrots, peeled and diced
2-3 celery stalks, sliced
12 teaspoons olive oil
½ teaspoon salt
½ teaspoon pepper
4-6 cups vegetable broth, chicken broth, or miso broth (3/4 cup miso paste mixed with 4-5 cups warm water)

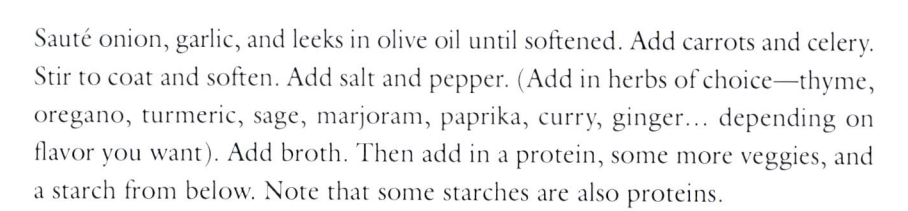

Sauté onion, garlic, and leeks in olive oil until softened. Add carrots and celery. Stir to coat and soften. Add salt and pepper. (Add in herbs of choice—thyme, oregano, turmeric, sage, marjoram, paprika, curry, ginger... depending on flavor you want). Add broth. Then add in a protein, some more veggies, and a starch from below. Note that some starches are also proteins.

Protein: Beans, lentils, sausage, tofu, cooked chicken, left over meat, shrimp, fish, clams, crab.

Vegetables: Spinach, kale, squash, green beans, swiss chard, parsnips, tomato, zucchini

Starch: wild rice, barley, faro, tortellini, orzo, spelt, potato, sweet potato, beans, lentils

• • •

Southwestern Seafood Corn Chowder
1 teaspoon olive oil
1 leek, sliced
1-2 shallots, chopped
1 medium carrot, peeled and chopped
1 roasted red pepper, diced (roast whole pepper in oven at 350 degrees for

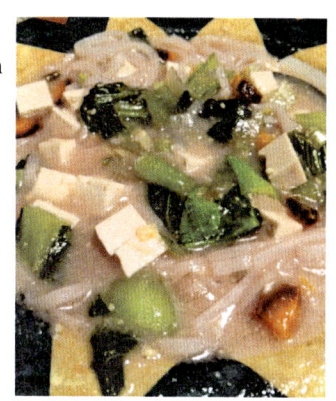

ten to fifteen minutes)
½ teaspoon chili powder
1 teaspoon cumin
½ teaspoon oregano
Pinch of sea salt
3 grinds pepper (add cayenne pepper, if you like heat)
1-2 new potatoes, cleaned and cubed (can use sweet potato instead)
1-2 cups organic corn kernels, fresh or frozen.
4 cups of vegetable or chicken broth, low sodium.
1 cup of milk of choice (cow, goat, almond, coconut milk)
1-2 cup lump crab meat (real not imitation) or wild, sustainable salmon, cooked

In a Dutch oven pan, heat olive oil, sauté shallots, and leeks until softening. Add carrots and cook about one minute to soften. Add in chopped red pepper, chili, cumin, oregano, salt, and pepper. Mix in vegetables and coat in herbs/seasoning. Pour in the broth and milk, and heat on medium high to bring to low boil. Add in the potatoes and corn. Mix and cook about five to eight minutes. Mix in the seafood of choice. If it is not yet cooked, add in and cook for another eight to ten minutes. Serve soup in bowls, optionally topping with chopped cilantro and/or tortilla strips.

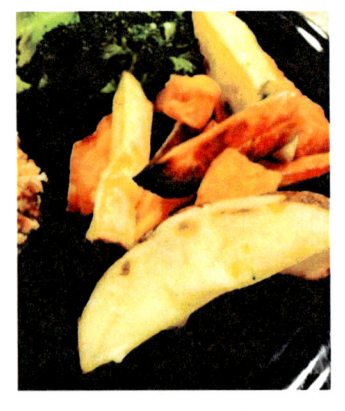

• • •

Sweet Potato Fries
2 medium sweet potatoes, peeled and sliced into 1 inch wedges
1 teaspoon extra virgin olive oil (EVOO)
½ teaspoon sea salt
2-3 grinds of pepper

Arrange wedges on a baking sheet, and toss with EVOO, salt, and pepper. Bake at 325 degrees for twenty to twenty-five minutes, until browned and crispy.

• • •

Roasted Root Vegetables

1 delicata or acorn squash, peeled and diced
1 sweet potato diced
1 parsnip or carrot diced

Toss in olive oil with sprinkle of salt on baking sheet. Cook 400 degrees, tossing half way, for twenty to thirty minutes until browned.

. . .

Roasted Brussel Sprouts

2-4 cups Brussel sprouts, rinsed and halved
1-2 tablespoons extra virgin olive oil
1 teaspoon sea salt

Place halved Brussel sprouts on baking sheet. Toss with olive oil and sea salt. Bake at 400 degrees for fifteen to twenty minutes, tossing half way to evenly roast. They should be browned and slightly crispy.

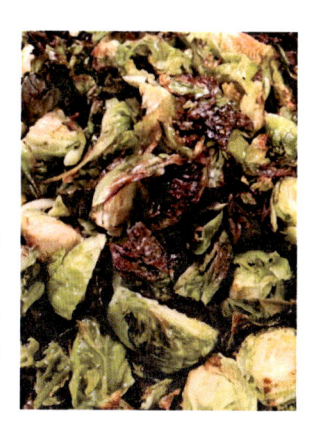

. . .

Southwestern 'Caviar'

1 firm, ripe avocado diced
2-3 Roma or heirloom tomatoes, diced
4 green onions, rinsed and sliced
1-2 ears of leftover corn, cut off the cob
1 16 ounce can of BPA free black beans, drained and rinsed
1 clove garlic, minced
2 tablespoon red wine vinegar
1 ½ tablespoon olive oil or grapeseed oil
1 teaspoon ground cumin
¼ cup chopped fresh cilantro
1 teaspoon lime juice
½ teaspoon salt
Dash of pepper

* if you like spicy, add 1 teaspoon of hot sauce or cayenne pepper
1 can of rinsed and drained organic black beans
Mix it all up and serve as a side, as a hearty summer salad or as a snack with tortilla chips. Delish!

• • •

Baked Kale Chips*

4 cups kale, rinsed
1-2 tablespoon extra-virgin olive oil
1 teaspoon sea salt

Rinse kale leaves, pat dry, and rip into chunky pieces off the stems. Place on cookie sheet, toss with 1-2 tablespoons EVOO and a pinch of salt. Bake at 375 degrees for five to eight minutes, until crispy, but not burnt. Toss ½ way to roast evenly. Eat them just like chips!!

• • •

Beet Chips

2-3 Beets of your choice, golden, red, bull's eye or assorted.

Peel beets then slice in rounds thinly with knife, vegetable peeler, or ideally, with a mandolin, about ⅛ - ¼ inch thick. Rinse beet rounds under cold water until they stop "bleeding" (color not as bright). Pat dry.

You can eat as chips, or dip in dressing. OR…

Beat a ¼ cup of goat cheese to soften, then spoon into a plastic bag. Squish the goat cheese into a corner, snip the corner off of the bag below cheese. Squeeze goat cheese into quarter sized dollops onto beet round. This is a great appetizer or snack.

• • •

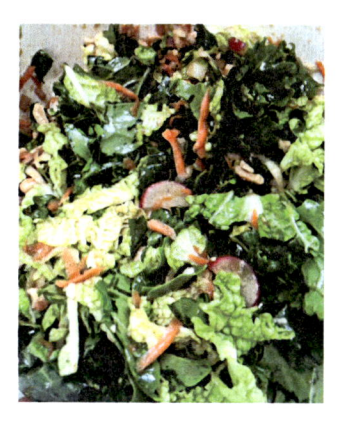

Asian Kale Salad

2-4 cups kale, rinsed and pulled off the stems
1 shallot, diced
¼ cup sesame oil
¼ cup soy sauce
1 teaspoon honey
½ cup chopped cashews
Optional: 1 cup red cabbage, diced and/or chopped Brussel sprouts added to kale

Chop the kale into small chunks, and place in a bowl. Mix shallots, sesame oil, soy sauce, and honey in a small bowl. Pour over the kale, and with your hands, massage the dressing into the kale to loosen and break up the tough kale fibers. Mix in the cashews. Let it sit for thirty minutes or more, and serve as main dish or side.

• • •

Broccoli or Green Beans in Lemon Oil

2-3 cups of broccoli florrettes, broccolini, or green beans, steamed to gentle softening (2-3 minutes steamed max)
2 tablespoons olive oil
2 tablespoons fresh lemon juice
1 teaspoon lemon zest
Pinch of salt and pepper

Mix steamed veggies in lemon oil.

Chapter 8

Main Meals

"The only real stumbling block is fear of failure. In cooking, you've got to have a what-the-hell attitude." - Julia Child

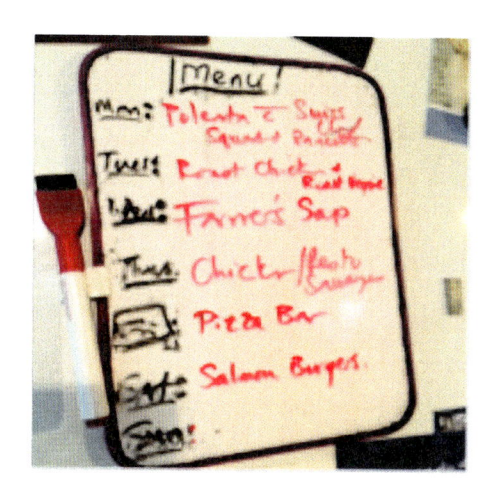

Cashew Chicken
4 skinless, boneless chicken breast, diced
1-2 tablespoons cornstarch
Salt and pepper
1 head of broccoli, rinsed and chopped
4-6 green onions, diced
3 cloves garlic, minced
1 red pepper
¼ cup hoisin sauce (or ¼ cup soy sauce, 1 teaspoon garlic, 1-2 tablespoons honey, 1 teaspoon sesame oil)
¼ cup water
½ cup unsalted, roasted cashews
1 cup brown rice, rinsed and cooked as directed

Coat chicken in cornstarch, salt, and pepper. Brown chicken in a sauté pan with 1-2 teaspoons sesame or olive oil. Cook chicken in batches until browned and cooked through. Remove chicken to a plate.

Next, sauté garlic, broccoli, and red pepper until softened. Add chicken back to pan, then add hoisin sauce and water. Mix, and cook for one to two minutes until broccoli is softened and liquid begins to thicken. Add cashews. Stir to mix. Spoon chicken mixture over rice to serve.

• • •

Jen's Yummy Turkey Burgers
1 pound lean ground turkey
1 cup grated carrots (about 2-3)
1 cup grated zucchini (1 big or 2 small)
1 small diced onion (sautéed in EVOO)
1 cup chopped spinach (fresh or frozen)
¼ cup grated parmesan
4 tablespoons Worcestershire sauce
(1 egg white if not binding)

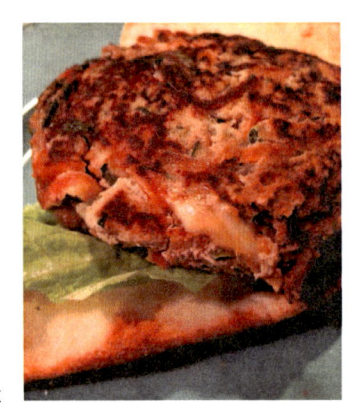

Combine ingredients in a large bowl, and mix well with hands until blended. Make into 3 ounce patties, about the size of the palm of your hand. Cook on griddle if using the stovetop, or grill on BBQ (on tinfoil) until browned and firm to touch. Serve on a whole grain roll, pita, or English muffin with homemade sweet potato fries

• • •

Tolo's Turkey Meatballs (or Meatloaf)
1 pound ground turkey
1 cup grated carrots
1 cup grated zucchini
½ cup grated parmesan
1 ½ teaspoon oregano,
1 teaspoon basil

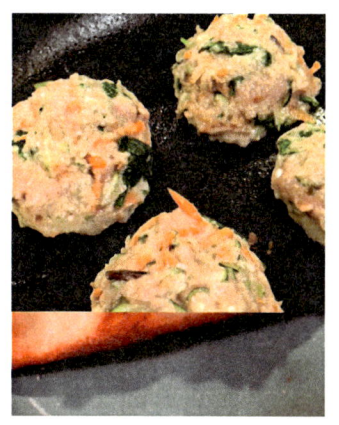

¾ cup panko breadcrumbs
1 egg white
Mix ingredients thoroughly in large bowl to distribute ingredients evenly. Roll meat mixture into golf ball size or smaller. Place on parchment or tinfoil lined baking sheet. Broil in oven ten to fifteen minutes, turning meatballs halfway through cooking process. Cook until browned.

For sauce, simmer one 32 ounce can of crushed tomatoes in saucepan, adding: 1 teaspoon oregano, 1 teaspoon basil and a pinch of salt and pepper. Add meatballs to heat through, and serve over pasta or polenta.

You can save meatballs out of sauce to put in a soup, or make meatball sandwiches, or put on homemade pizza. It is good to make a big batch.

NOTE: If making meatloaf, press meat mixture in loaf pan, top with BBQ sauce and ketchup (1 tablespoon each) bake for forty-five minutes at 350 degrees. You can make mini loafs too forming on a cookie sheet, palm size.

Note: You can make your own breadcrumbs, even GF. Take your favorite bread (I like Trader Joes quinoa bread and use ends of the loaf), pulse in Cuisinart with herbs. Put in sealable container and keep in fridge or freezer.

. . .

Bolognese or Meat Sauce
1 pound ground turkey
1 cup carrots, grated
1 cup zucchini, grated
1 small onion, diced
1 clove garlic
1 red bell pepper diced

32 ounce can of crushed tomatoes
½ teaspoon fennel
1 teaspoon basil
1 teaspoon oregano
¼ cup fresh grated parmesan

Brown the ground meat. Drain excess liquid, and reserve meat. Sauté onion and garlic in olive oil (1-2 teaspoons) over medium heat. Add bell peppers, grated zucchini, and carrots. Mix well, and add crushed tomato and browned meat. Mix well. Add in salt, pepper, fennel, basil, and oregano. Mix well, and simmer on low for ten minutes, then add ¼ grated parmesan to sauce and serve over pasta, polenta, or spaghetti squash.

• • •

Bonus meal: TURKEY CHILI
Use same ingredients and process, but add these spice substitutions and one can of red kidney beans, rinsed and drained. Simmer for fifteen to twenty minutes.

Spice Changes:
2 teaspoons cumin
2-4 tablespoons ground chili
1 teaspoon oregano

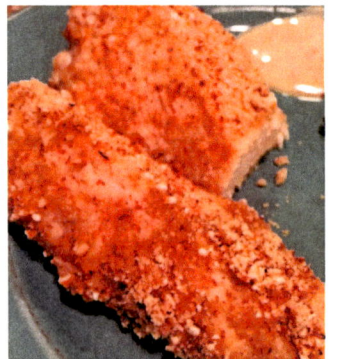

• • •

Almond Chicken Tenders or Cutlets
4-6 chicken cutlets, cut in about 3-4 ounce pieces
1 cup roasted unsalted almond
Optional: ½ cup whole grain, multi-grain, or gluten free pretzels.

Place almonds and, if you choose, pretzels into a food processor. Grind into a coarse flour. Pour mixture into a shallow bowl. Place chicken cutlets or tenders (you can cut cutlets into strips for tenders) into flour mixture. Coat the chicken in the flour mixture, covering all sides. Place on an olive oil sprayed baking sheet. Bake at 375 degrees for twenty to twenty-five minutes until chicken is slightly browned and firm to touch.

*I like to serve these with sweet potato fries or roasted root vegetables and either steamed broccoli or roasted Brussel sprouts.

• • •

Macaroni and Cheese Change Up

1 box pasta of choice
2 tablespoons butter
2 tablespoons flour
1 cup milk (skim or 1%)
1 ½ cups shredded cheddar cheese
1 teaspoon ground mustard
1-2 cups of diced tomatoes, steamed and mashed cauliflower, or roasted and mashed butternut squash

Boil pasta. While pasta is boiling, in a medium saucepan, melt butter and add flour. Mix flour and butter to make a roux. Add milk and ground mustard. Add cheese, and stir to smooth consistency. Add boiled pasta and sauce together. Mix to coat pasta with sauce. Add your vegetable of choice, and mix well. Serve as is, or for crunchier mac'n'cheese, bake at 350 degrees for ten minutes.

Note: Gluten Free options can be with GF Pasta (rice or corn/quinoa or with veggies like spaghetti squash and/or zucchini ribbons.

• • •

Asian Chicken and Lettuce Wraps

pound ground turkey or chicken, browned
1-2 diced or shredded carrots
1 zucchini, shredded
1 shallot, diced
2 cups spinach, rinsed and dried.

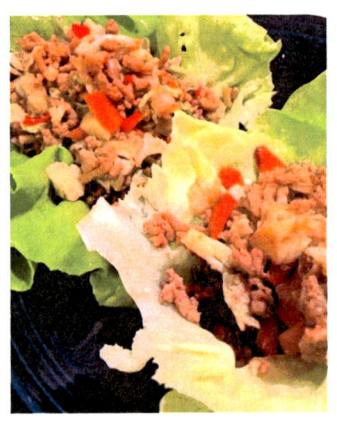

1 cup cabbage of choice (Napa, red or green)
3-4 tablespoons hoisin sauce
1 tsp sesame oil
A head of Bibb, Boston, or red/green leaf lettuce, rinsed and dried.

Sauté shallots in sesame oil. Add browned turkey, carrots, zucchini, spinach, and cabbage. Mix and heat gently. Add hoisin sauce and 1 tablespoon of water to thin sauce. Mix well. Spoon into lettuce leafs. Wrap up and enjoy.

CAUTION: It can get messy…

Note: You can add brown rice to wraps as well or pine nuts or almonds for flavor.

• • •

Simple Spanish Rice, Spinach and Chick Peas

1-2 shallots, diced
1 package or 4 cups baby spinach, rinsed
2 cloves garlic, minced
1 can BPA free chickpeas, drained and rinsed
1 ½ teaspoon cumin
1 teaspoon Paprika or Cayenne Pepper
2-3 cups cooked brown rice

Sauté shallots, garlic, and spinach in 1teaspoon of EVOO. Add a can of rinsed chickpeas. Add 2-3 cups precooked brown rice, 1 ½ teaspoon cumin, and 1 teaspoon paprika or cayenne pepper (depending on your taste, spicey or smokey).

Spoon it up, and enjoy for lunch or dinner as a meal or with a side of meat.
Note: This is a great meal/side for a family with some carnivores and some vegetarians.

Coconut Crusted Haddock

2 pounds haddock, cut into 4 pieces (you can use cod as well)
1 cup coconut milk
1 teaspoon chili powder
½ teaspoon cinnamon
1 tablespoon lime juice
1 tablespoon cilantro
1 cup shredded coconut (unsweetened and fine is best)

Soak fish in coconut milk, lime juice, chili, cinnamon, and cilantro mixture for two to three minutes. Remove fish from coconut milk mixture and roll to cover it in coconut. Heat 2 tablespoons olive or sesame oil in pan. Fry fish, cooking over medium heat for two minutes a side or until browned and heated through. You want the fish to be firm to the touch and flakey. You can serve as fish tacos or as side to quinoa pilaf.

• • •

Quinoa Pilaf (Serve with Coconut Fish) *can do with faro/orzo/rice

1 cup of quinoa (cooked in 2 cups chicken or vegetable broth)
¼ cup slivered almonds
2 cups fresh baby spinach chopped, or 1 box of frozen organic spinach
1 tablespoon chopped cilantro
1 teaspoon cumin
2 clementines/mandarin oranges

Add the slivered almonds and spinach to the cooked quinoa. Toss in the cilantro and cumin. Mix well. Peel and juice one clementine over quinoa and one over fish, then section remaining parts and mix in with quinoa.

• • •

Salmon Burgers

1-2 pounds wild caught salmon, deboned and skinned (Do not us farm raised salmon, as its high in toxins)
1 slice of whole wheat bread, grinded in food processor
1 tablespoon fresh grated ginger
2 tablespoons grainy Dijon mustard
3 green onions diced, whites only

Place all ingredients in a food processor and blend to mix. Scoop out ½-1 cup portions and form into patties. Place on wax paper lined plate. Make six to eight patties. Pan sear like a burger. Serve alone or on whole grain bun, English muffin, or oat bran pita. (You can freeze extra patties.)

Sesame Lime Mayonnaise: Start with ¼ cup mayonnaise (I like Helman's Olive Oil), add 1 teaspoon sesame oil, and 1 teaspoon lime juice. Top salmon burgers with a one to two teaspoons of this for more flavor.

• • •

Tuscan Chicken

1 pound boneless, skinless chicken thighs
4 cups rinsed, chopped kale
1 can cannellini beans, drained and rinsed
2 large shallots, diced
1 leek, diced and rinsed
2 large carrots, peeled and diced
2 tablespoons rosemary
2 cloves garlic, minced
1 cup dry white wine (like Pinot Grigio)
¼ cup olive oil
½ cup chicken broth
1 cup faro or wild rice cooked in 2 cups chicken broth

Sauté shallots, 1 clove garlic, leeks, and carrots in large sauce pan with olive oil until softened. Place chicken in pan, top with 1 ½ teaspoon rosemary, salt, and pepper. Brown chicken, turning over in pan several times. Add chicken broth, beans, and kale. Simmer for five to eight minutes until liquid is reduced in pan.

Heat wine and remaining rosemary in small saucepan. In food processor, place oil, garlic, and wine infusion. Blend to a sauce consistency. Add sauce mixture to chicken, and simmer for five minutes. Place chicken on top of faro or rice to serve.

• • •

Veg-Out Eggplant Parmesan Casserole: *(Meatless Mondays)*

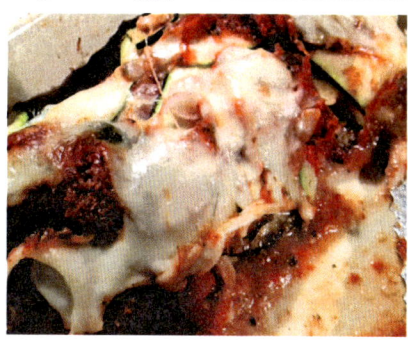

1 large or 2 small eggplants, sliced ¼ inch thick in rounds (*Step Saver: buy frozen cutlets at Trader Joes*)
1 egg
1 cup panko bread crumbs or spelt flour, or mix
1 teaspoon oregano
1 teaspoon basil
1 tube polenta, sliced in ¼ inch rounds
1-2 zucchini, sliced in rounds or lengthwise, thin
2-3 tomatoes, sliced in rounds
1 red onion, sliced in thin rounds
2 cups of tomato sauce (fresh or prepared)
½ cup grated parmesan
1 fresh ball of mozzarella, sliced ¼ inch rounds

Step 1: Prepare eggplant cutlets. Lightly salt cutlets, let sit between paper towels for five minutes. Rinse and pat dry. Combine bread crumbs, or flour, oregano, basil and ¼ cup parmesan in shallow bowl. Whisk egg in shallow bowl. Dredge eggplant cutlet in egg, then flour/breadcrumb. Fry in a pan over medium heat with 1-2 tablespoons extra virgin olive oil. Set aside on plate with paper towel to drain.

Step 2: In casserole or lasagna pan, layer sauce, polenta, eggplant, onion, zucchini, then tomato. Top with sauce and cheese and repeat layer. Top with sauce, grated parmesan, and mozzarella. Bake at 350 degrees for twenty-five to thirty minutes.

• • •

B-Man's Peanut Noodles

½ cup peanut butter (smooth, natural with no added sugar)
¼ cup soy sauce
⅛ cup warm water
1 tablespoon fresh grated ginger
1 clove garlic minced
2 tablespoons sesame oil
2 tablespoons honey
1 ½ tablespoons rice wine vinegar
1 cup chopped cabbage (we like Napa)
1 cup diced or shredded carrots
1 cup chopped broccoli
1 cup chopped spinach or Bok Choy
4-6 scallions, diced
8 ounces rice stick noodles or soba noodles (buckwheat noodles)

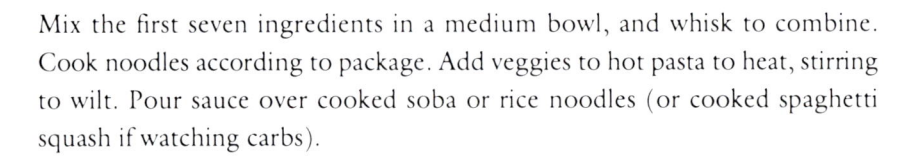

Mix the first seven ingredients in a medium bowl, and whisk to combine. Cook noodles according to package. Add veggies to hot pasta to heat, stirring to wilt. Pour sauce over cooked soba or rice noodles (or cooked spaghetti squash if watching carbs).

Note: You can make sauce and ready veggies ahead of time and keep in fridge for six to eight hours. This is a time saver.

Note: Rice noodles are sticky and less flavorful while soba noodles are firmer with a nutty flavor and more nutrients.

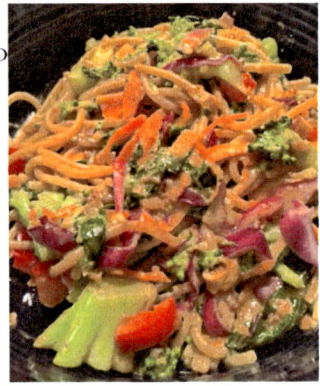

Chapter 9

Marvelous Muffins

I love to make muffins. In fact, many of my friends have dubbed me "the muffin lady," as I am always sharing my muffins or my recipes. I love to make healthy, nutrient rich, grab and go foods for my busy family, so they do not skip breakfast. My husband will often grab a few muffins on his way out the door in the morning and so will my boys, who like to sleep as late as they can and need to run out the door to catch the bus. My family likes the muffins as their snack as well.

I hope you enjoy these yummy, healthy bites. Please note that the whole wheat flour and spelt or oat flour will make these denser and less "fluffy," but they are more nutrient rich and still moist. I use spelt flour in my muffins, as it is easier to digest and high in zinc.

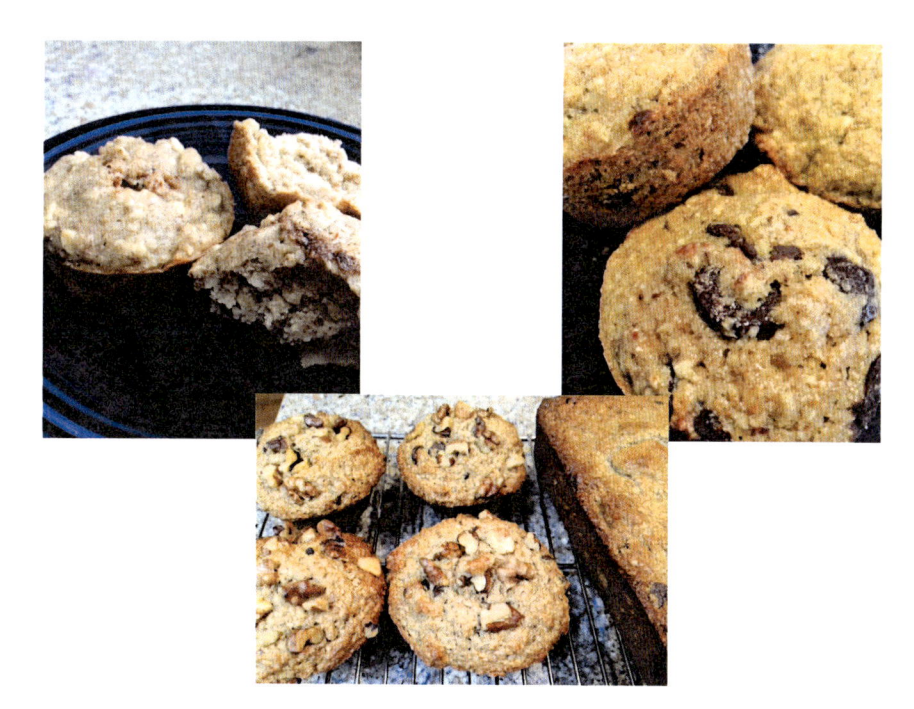

Banana Bran Muffins (makes 12- 16 muffins)
1¼ cups oat flour
1 cup oat bran
2 tablespoons ground flaxseed (Omega 3)
1 teaspoon baking powder
½ teaspoon salt
2-3 mashed ripe bananas (I use my over- ripe bananas the kids won't eat)
½ cup coconut oil, heated over low heat, or sunflower oil
½ cup organic brown sugar or maple syrup
1 teaspoon vanilla
1 egg
Optional: ½ cup walnuts, ½ cup dark chocolate chips.
Add 1-2 tablespoons milk to thin batter to spoon into greased muffin tins.

Combine flour, oat bran, flaxseed, baking powder, and salt in small bowl. Set it aside. Mix together the sugar, oil, bananas, and vanilla. Beat in the egg. Add the dry ingredients to the wet ingredients. Fold in chocolate chips and/or walnuts. Spoon into greased muffin tins, filling three-quarters of the way full. Bake at 350 degrees for eighteen to twenty minutes.

• • •

Strawberry Cream Muffins (makes 12-16 muffins)
1 cup organic strawberries, rinsed and quartered
1 squeeze of lemon juice
1¼ cups oat flour (for gluten free), or 1 cup whole wheat pastry flour
½ cup whole oats
1 teaspoon baking powder
½ teaspoon salt
⅓ cup maple syrup
¼ cup coconut oil (heated gently just to liquid.)
½ cup plain greek yogurt
1 teaspoon vanilla extract
1 large egg

Squeeze lemon over sliced strawberries and coat. Mix flour, oats, baking powder, and salt in a medium bowl. Combine maple syrup, coconut oil, greek yogurt, and vanilla in a large bowl. Stir to combine. Beat in the egg. Add wet ingredients to dry ingredients, mixing well. Fold in strawberries. Spoon into lightly greased (sprayed) muffin tins. Makes twelve to sixteen muffins. Bake at 400 degrees for fifteen minutes

• • •

Blueberry Oat Muffins (12-16 muffins)
1½ cups whole wheat pastry flour or spelt flour
½ cup quick cook oats
2 teaspoons baking powder
½ teaspoon baking powder
½ teaspoon salt
⅓ cup sugar or maple syrup
¾ cup plain Greek yogurt (or silken tofu, if dairy free)
¼ cup applesauce
¼ cup coconut oil, heated to liquid over low heat, or sunflower oil
1 egg
1 teaspoon vanilla
1¼ cups fresh or frozen organic blueberries
2-4 tablespoons milk to thin out batter
Optional: ¼ cup slivered almonds for tops

Preheat oven to 375 degrees. Spray muffin tins with cooking spray (olive or coconut oil). Mix flour, oats, baking powder, baking soda, and salt in a large bowl. Mix sugar, yogurt, applesauce, and coconut oil in medium bowl. Beat in egg and vanilla. Add wet ingredients to dry, stirring just enough to mix. Fold in blueberries. Add enough milk to thin batter to pourable consistency. Spoon into muffin tins, and top with almonds. Bake at 375 degrees for eighteen to twenty minutes.

• • •

Crunchy Pumpkin Muffins
(makes 16-20 muffins or 1 loaf and 6 muffins)
½ cup raw pepitas or pumpkin seeds (toasted in oven at 400 degrees for five to eight minutes)

2 cups whole wheat pastry, spelt, or oat flour
1 teaspoon baking powder
¾ teaspoon allspice
½ teaspoon salt
½ cup brown sugar or date sugar
¼ cup honey
¾ cup pure pumpkin puree
¼ cup coconut oil, heated to liquid over low heat
¼ cup applesauce
1 teaspoon vanilla
2 eggs
2-4 tablespoons milk to thin out batter

Preheat oven to 375 degrees. Spray muffin tins with coconut or olive oil spray. Mix flour, baking powder, allspice, and salt in medium bowl. In large bowl, mix sugar, pumpkin purée, honey, coconut oil, applesauce, and vanilla. Beat in eggs one at a time. Add dry ingredients to wet, mixing well in batches. Add milk as needed to thin out batter to pourable or spoonable consistency. Fold in pumpkin seeds, or top muffins with seeds. Spoon batter into tins. Bake at 375 degrees for eighteen to twenty minutes.

• • •

Apple Oat Spice Muffins
⅓ cup spelt flour (high in zinc)
1 cup quick cook oats
½ cup oat flour
¼ cup ground flaxseed (omega 3)
1 teaspoon baking powder
½ teaspoon baking soda
¼ teaspoon sea salt
1 teaspoon cinnamon
½ teaspoon nutmeg
¼ teaspoon cardamom
⅛ teaspoon ground ginger
1 cup applesauce, unsweetened
½ cup plain yogurt

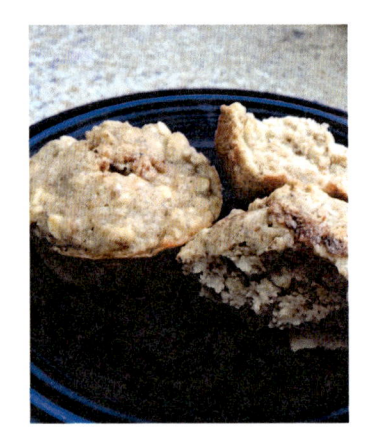

½ cup pure maple syrup
3 tablespoons coconut oil, heated to liquid
2 tablespoons apple cider
1 egg beaten
1 teaspoon vanilla
2 apples, your choice, roughly peeled, some skin on, cored and diced

Preheat oven 375 degrees. Grease or spray twelve to eighteen muffin tins (I baked these on a dozen regular size muffin tin and on a one dozen mini-muffin tin.)

Combine dry ingredients in large bowl. Stir to mix. Combine wet ingredients in a large bowl, mix well, then slowly mix in the dry ingredients. Finally, fold in the apple chunks and nuts, if you choose. Pour batter into muffin tins, and bake at 375 for twenty to twenty-three minutes.

Chapter 10

Delicious Desserts

"All you need is love. But a little chocolate now and then doesn't hurt"
-Charles M. Schultz

Apple Cake
1½ cup whole wheat pastry, spelt or oat flour
¾ cup oats
1 teaspoon baking soda
½ teaspoon cinnamon
½ teaspoon cardamom
½ teaspoon salt
½ cup brown sugar, date sugar or Maple Syrup (pure)
¼ cup coconut oil, heated to liquid on low
¼ cup safflower or sunflower oil
1 cup plain Greek yogurt
½ cup buttermilk
½ cup applesauce
1 egg
1 cup peeled and diced apples
1 cup confectioner's sugar to sift on top

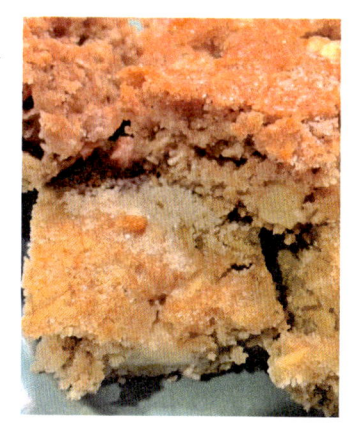

Preheat oven to 350 degrees. Line a nine-inch round or eight-by-eight-inch pan with parchment paper, and spray with cooking spray. In large bowl, mix together flour, oats, spices, salt, and baking soda. In medium bowl, mix oil, applesauce, yogurt and sugar. Beat in one egg and apple cider. Add the wet ingredients to the dry, stirring to mix. Fold in apple chinks. Pour batter into lined pan. Bake at 350 degrees for forty to forty-five minutes, until edges are browned and cake springs back to touch. Sift confectioner's sugar to dust the top and serve.

Jennifer Wren Tolo, RN

• • •

"Butterflied" CARROT CAKE MUFFINS or CAKE

4 eggs
¼ cups coconut oil, heated to liquid over low heat
¼ cup safflower oil
¼ cup applesauce
¾ cup turbanado or raw sugar
½ cup honey
1 teaspoon vanilla
2 cups whole wheat pastry flour, spelt flour, or (for GF) 2 1/2 cups oat flour
2 teaspoons baking soda
½ teaspoon salt
2 teaspoons baking powder
1 teaspoon ground ginger
2 teaspoons ground cinnamon
3 cups grated carrots
1 cup chopped walnuts

Mix oil, sugar, applesauce, and honey in large bowl. Add vanilla, and beat in eggs. Mix to combine. In medium bowl, mix flour, baking powder and soda, salt, ginger, and cinnamon. Slowly, in stages, add dry ingredients to wet, and mix to combine. Add grated carrots and walnuts, mixing well. Pour into greased muffin tins or nine-by-nine-inch baking pan for cake. Bake at 350 degrees for twenty-five minutes, or until springy to touch.

• • •

Cream Cheese Frosting:
4 tablespoons butter, softened (I like Kerrigold or Kate's)
8 ounces softened cream cheese (I like the Greek yogurt cream cheese)
1 cup honey
½ cup to 1 cup confectioner's sugar (depends on consistency)
1 teaspoon vanilla

Blend with mixer and spread over cooled cupcakes or cake.

Peanut Butter Chocolate Chip Bites

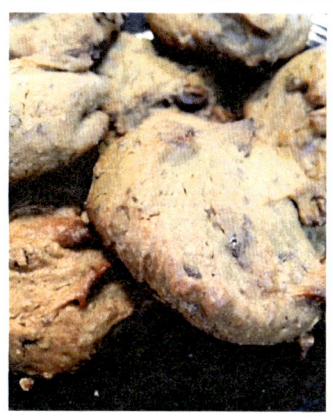

1 cup smooth peanut butter
½ cup honey
¼ cup ground flaxseed
1 egg
½ cup dark chocolate chips (Ghirdelli 60% Cacoa)

Mix and drop by spoonful on cookie sheet. Bake 350 degrees for ten minutes. Makes ten to twelve bites.

• • •

Chocolate Cherry Bombs

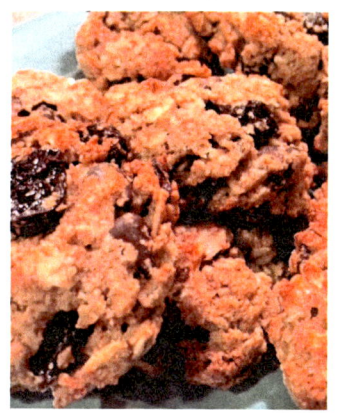

¾ cup whole wheat flour, spelt flour or oat flour (They will be dense.)
½ cup rolled oats
½ teaspoon baking soda
½ teaspoon salt
½ teaspoon cinnamon
¼ cup safflower oil
¼ cup applesauce
⅛ cup brown sugar
2 tablespoons granulated sugar
1 egg
1 teaspoon vanilla
¼ tsp sea salt
¼ cup chopped walnuts
½ cup chocolate chips
¼ cup cherries

Preheat oven to 375 degrees. Mix dry ingredients in a bowl. Mix wet ingredients in mixing bowl. Add dry ingredients to wet. Stir to incorporate. Fold in chocolate chips, walnuts, and cherries. Drop onto cookie sheet using teaspoon or small ice cream scoop about two inches apart. Bake until golden brown, about eight to ten minutes.

• • •

Guilt Free Gooey Brownies (Gluten Free)
6 tablespoons coconut oil
12 ounces chocolate chips 1/3 cup cornstarch
2 tablespoons ground flaxseeds
¼ cup unsweetened cocoa
½ teaspoon cinnamon
½ teaspoon salt
½ cup maple syrup or raw honey
1 tsp vanilla
3 large eggs

Combine cornstarch, flaxseeds, unsweetened cocoa, cinnamon, and salt in a bowl and mix. In a saucepan, heat coconut oil and chocolate chips over medium to low heat. Remove chocolate mix from heat, and add maple syrup or honey, vanilla, and eggs. Add wet to dry ingredients and mix to incorporate. Pour into parchment lined, cooking sprayed pan, eight-by-ten or nine-by-nine inches. Bake at 350 degrees for twenty-five to thirty minutes. You can dust the top with confectioner's sugar, if you want.

• • •

Banana Boats (Great dessert or snack)

1 banana, sliced in half length-wise
1 tablespoon organic and natural peanut butter
1 tablespoon good quality granola
1 tablespoon chocolate chips

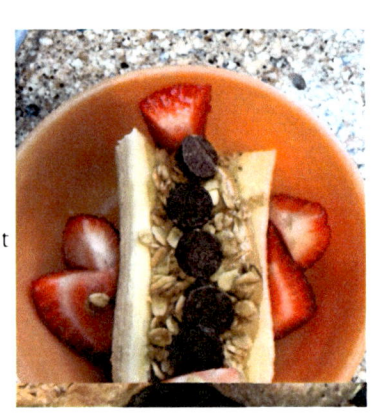

(For a really creamy treat, you can top with REAL whipped cream—no Cool Whip!)

In a bowl, butterfly the banana open. Spread peanut butter along the middle. Sprinkle granola and chocolate chips over the top. Top with whipped cream dollop or Greek yogurt.

. . .

Chocolate Fruit Fondue
¾ cup high quality chocolate chips (I like Ghiardelli's 60 percent cacao)
1 tablespoon coconut oil
1-2 cups assorted fruit (strawberries, cherries, apples, bananas, pears)

Heat the chocolate chips and butter in double boiler over gentle heat, and stir to melt chocolate. Place in bowl in center of a plate of assorted fruit. Dip fruit in chocolate mix. Delish!

. . .

Raw Chocolate Coconut Almond Bites of Joy (Makes 10-12 Bites)
1 cup unsweetened shredded coconut
¼ cup coconut oil
2 tablespoons pure maple syrup
1 teaspoon vanilla
12 raw almonds
Pinch of sea salt
1 cup dark chocolate chips (60 percent or more cacao)

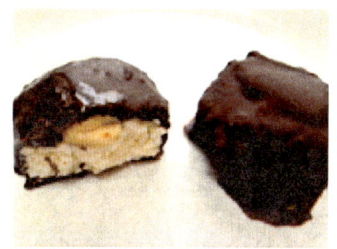

In a double boiler, or bowl over saucepan of boiling water, melt chocolate chips with teaspoon coconut oil. Be careful to not overheat, just melt chocolate. In a food processor, place coconut, oil, vanilla, maple syrup, and salt. Pulse to combine well. Line a cookie sheet with parchment or wax paper. Using a small melon baller or ice cream scoop, scoop out a tablespoon of the coconut mixture, forming a domed circle. Press an almond into top of dome. Gently lower the coconut ball into the chocolate, and using a spoon, cover the ball in chocolate. Carefully lift out and place on the parchment lined sheet. Repeat this process for all of the "balls of joy." Place in the freezer or refrigerator to solidify. You can serve cold or frozen. A great, sweet, crunchy, and creamy treat without the guilt or derailment of too much fat and sugar!

Resources

Albers, Susan. *Eating Mindfully: How to End Mindless Eating and Have a Relationship with Food.* 2012, www.newharbinger.com.

Behan, Eileen. *Fit Kids: Raising Physically and Emotionally Strong Kids with Real Food.* New York: Pocket Books, 2001.

Campbell, T. Colin, Jacobson, Howard. *Whole: Rethinking the Science of Nutrition.* Dallas, Texas: BenBella Books, 2013.

Chapman, C.D, et al. "Lifestyle Determinants of the Drive to Eat: A Meta-Analysis." *American Journal of Clinical Nutrition.* 2012: 96 (3), 492-97.

Crinnion, Walter. *Clean, Green and Lean.* Hoboken, NJ: John Wiley & Sons, 2010.

Davis, Willam, MD. *The Wheat Belly Diet.* New York: Rodale, 2011.

DGAC (Dietary Guidelines Advisory Committee). *Scientific Report of the 2015 Dietary Guidelines Advisory Committee.* 2015, http://health.gov/dietaryguidlines/2015-scientific-report/PDFs/Scientific-Report-of-the-2015-Dietary-Guidelines-Advisory-Committee.pdf.

Doulliard, John. *Three Season Diet: Solving Mysterious Food Cravings, Weight Loss and Exercise.* Berkley, CA: North Atlantic Books, 2000.

Fides, A., van Jaarsveld, C., Llewellyn, C., Fisher, A., Cooke, L., Wardle, J. "Nature and Nurture in Children's Food Preferences." *The American Journal of Clinical Nutrition.* 2014: 99:911-917.

Geagan, Kate. *Go Green, Get Lean.* New York: Rodale, 2009.

Hartman Group. "Snacking Our Way Through the Day: Food Culture in America." *Hartbeat, Newsletter of the Hartman Group.* 2004, http://hartbeat.hartman-group.com/article/64/.

Hartman Group. "Snacking in America Infographic." *Hartbeat, Newsletter of the Hartman Group.* 2013, http://hartbeat.hartman-group.com/article/457/Snacking-in-America-Infographic.

Kabat-Zinn, John. *Full Catastrophe Living: Using the Wisdom of Your Body and Mind to Face Stress, Pain and Illness.* New York: Delacorte, 2003.

Katz, David, MD. *Disease Proof: The Remarkable Truth About What Makes Us Well.* New York: Hudson Street Press, 2013.

Millar, Amy Myrdal. "Snack Attack: What's Up with the U.S. Snacking Obsession?" *IDEA Food and Nutrition Tips.* November-December 2015, 6-12.

Nestle, Marion. *What to Eat.* New York: North Point Press, 2006.

Owen, N., Bauman, A., Brown, W. "Too Much Sitting: A Novel and Important Predictor of Chronic Disease Risk?" *British Journal of Sports Medicine.* 2009: 43(2), 81-83.

Pearson, Natalie, and Biddle, Stuart. "Sedentary Behavior and Dietary Intake in Children, Adolescents and Adults." *American Journal of Preventative Medicine.* 2011, 41: 178-188.

Pederson, BK. "The Diseasome of Physical Inactivity—and the Role of Myokines in Muscle-Fat Cross Talk." *Journal of Physiology.* 2009: 587 (23), 5559-5568.

Pearson, Natalie. "Sedentary Behavior and Dietary Intake in Children, Adolescents, and Adults." *American Journal of Preventative Medicine.* August 2011: (41) 178-188.

Perlmutter, David, MD. *Grain Brain: The Surprising Truth About Wheat, Carbs and Sugar-your Brain's Silent Killers.* New York: Little, Brown and

Company, 2013.

Pollan, Micheal. *Food Rules: An Eater's Manual.* New York: Penguin Press, 2011.

Pollan, Micheal. *The Omnivore's Dilemma.* New York: Penguin Press, 2009.

Rao, M., Afshin, A., Singh, G., Motzaffarian, D. "Do Healthier Foods and Diet Patterns Cost More than Less Healthy Options? A Systematic Review and Meta-Analysis." *BMJ Open.* 2013.

Rosenthal, Joshua. *Integrative Nutrition.* Austin, Texas: Greenleaf Book Group, LLC, 2007.

Scaglioni, S., Arrizza, C., Vecchi, F., Tedeschi, S. "Determinants of Children's Eating Behavior." *The American Journal of Clinical Nutrition.* 2011, 94:2006S-2011S.

Sears, Willam, M.D. and Sears, Martha, R.N. *The Family Nutrition Book.* New York: Little, Brown and Company, 1999.

Somer, Elizabeth. *Food and Mood: The Complete Guide to Eating Well and Feeling Your Best.* New York: Henry Holt & Co, 1995, 1999.

L.H, Squirres, S. *The Stoplight Diet for Children.* Boston: Little, Brown and Company, 1988.

www.drweil.com

www.drhyman.com

www.feingold.org